Band 14, Supplement 2,
Dezember 2007

Offizielles Organ der Schweizerischen Medizinischen Gesellschaft für Phytotherapie
Offizielles Organ der Deutschen Gesellschaft für Naturheilkunde

Forschende Komplementärmedizin

Wissenschaft • Praxis • Perspektiven

Research in Complementary Medicine

Research • Practice • Perspectives

Informationen, Anfragen bitte direkt an:
S. Karger Verlag für Medizin
und Naturwissenschaften GmbH
Dipl. Psych. Franziska Lang
Lörracher Straße 16a
D-79115 Freiburg
f.lang@karger.de

KARGER

Basel · Freiburg · Paris · London · New York ·
Bangalore · Bangkok · Singapore · Tokyo · Sydney

Impressum

Die Zeitschrift erscheint zweimonatlich; pro Jahr erscheint 1 Band zu je 6 Heften. Bezugspreis für Jahrgang 14, 2007: Print-Abonnement EUR 164,–, Online-Abonnement EUR 164,–, Kombi-Abonnement Print/Online EUR 208,–, einschließlich MWSt., zuzüglich Postgebühren. Der Abonnementpreis ist im Voraus zahlbar. Das Abonnement der Zeitschrift läuft weiter, wenn es nicht spätestens 4 Wochen vor Abschluss eines Bandes abbestellt wird. Abonnementbestellungen können bei jeder Buchhandlung oder direkt beim Verlag aufgegeben werden:

Deutschland:
S. Karger Verlag für Medizin und Naturwissenschaften GmbH
Lörracher Str. 16a
D-79115 Freiburg
Tel. +49 761 45 20 70
Fax +49 761 4 52 07 14
E-mail Information@Karger.de

Übrige Länder:
S. Karger AG
Allschwilerstr. 10
Postfach
CH-4009 Basel
Tel. +41 61 3 06 11 11
Fax +41 61 3 06 12 34
E-mail Karger@Karger.ch

Anzeigen:
S. Karger Verlag für Medizin und Naturwissenschaften GmbH
Lörracher Str. 16a
D-79115 Freiburg,
Tel. +49 761 45 20 70
Gültig ist die Preisliste Nr. 10 vom 1. Januar 2007.

Supplement 2 zu Band 14, Dezember 2007
ISBN 978-3-8055-8503-3
e-ISBN 978-3-8055-8504-0

Verlagsleitung und presserechtlich verantwortlich: Sibylle Hopf
Produktionsleitung: Georg Brunner
Anzeigenleitung: Susanne Meister

Gesamtherstellung:
KONKORDIA GmbH, Bühl
Das Medienunternehmen

Bibliographische Dienste
Index Medicus/MEDLINE
Current Contents/Clinical Medicine
Science Citation Index Expanded
Index Copernicus

Forschende
Komplementärmedizin
Wissenschaft • Praxis • Perspektiven

Supplement 2,
Vol. 14,
December 2007

Medical Pluralism, Equity, Holism

Interdisciplinary Research Perspectives on Integrative Medicine

Editors

Florica Marian, Bern
Harald Walach, Northampton

KARGER

Basel · Freiburg · Paris · London · New York ·
Bangalore · Bangkok · Singapore · Tokyo · Sydney

Forschende Komplementärmedizin
Wissenschaft • Praxis • Perspektiven

Inhalt · Contents

Vol. 14, Supplement 2, Dezember 2007

Band 14, Supplement 2, December 2007

Peer Review: Jedes Manuskript wird von der Redaktion und von externen Gutachtern geprüft.

Peer Review: Each manuscript is evaluated by the editors and by external peer reviewers.

KARGER
Fax +49 761 4 52 07 14
E-mail Information@Karger.de
www.karger.com

Artikel (Volltext) und Inhaltsverzeichnisse sowie das vorläufige Inhaltsverzeichnis des nächsten Heftes:
www.karger.com/fok_bk.htm

Forschende Komplementärmedizin
Wissenschaft • Praxis • Perspektiven

Editorial

Forsch Komplementärmed 2007;14(suppl 2):1
DOI: 10.1159/000112494

Medical Pluralism, Equity and Holism

Florica Marian[a] Harald Walach[b]

[a] Institute for Complementary Medicine KIKOM, University of Bern, Switzerland
[b] University of Northampton, School of Social Sciences & Samueli Institute for Information Biology, Northampton, UK

Medical pluralism, equity and holism: these are research issues and perspectives arising in the Swiss Programme for the Evaluation of Complementary Medicine (PEK). This evaluation was commissioned by the Swiss Government in order to provide scientific data on 5 complementary therapies (anthroposophic medicine, homeopathy, neural therapy, phytotherapy and traditional Chinese medicine). The aim of PEK was to inform a policy decision about whether or not these disciplines, if provided by physicians in primary care, should be covered by basic health insurance. As PEK assessed a model of primary care which integrated conventional and complementary medicine – by comparing it with conventional primary care – I will also use the denomination 'integrative medicine'. PEK was carried out from 1998 to 2005. In that time, the government as well as the responsible authorities changed and decided against the definitive inclusion of the CAM methods in compulsory health coverage in June 2005. This was a political decision not supported by PEK data, and associated with a lack of fairness at several levels (e.g. exercise of political influence on the research process; the decision-making process itself). As equity and fairness are often neglected issues in the research literature on complementary and alternative medicine (CAM), they are investigated in two articles presented here. Holism, however, is very often mentioned and addressed in CAM research. The PEK data confirm the importance of holism as a core dimension for both physicians and patients. Moreover, they allow to include the aspect of physician satisfaction into a four-dimension model which comprises wholeness of patient, wholeness of physician, integration of therapeutic approaches and a relational dimension.

The thematic focus of this supplement is influenced by my own experience as a researcher participating in the PEK observational studies conducted in Swiss primary care and especially in the study on physicians' philosophy of care. Moreover, the daily confrontation with political and academic pressure and misuse of power motivated me to explore equity issues in more detail. My background in medical and cultural anthropology may also have contributed to a reflection on equity which takes into account both the role of the participant and the role of the observer. As a consequence, three methodological approaches are combined in the articles of this supplement: (1) an empirical approach, (2) a normative approach (a form of ethical enquiry and reflection on what should be or what a fair process would look like, and (3) a theoretical approach (discussing concepts of equity and holism). Such an interdisciplinary approach to both methodology and concerned fields, i.e. ethics, political science, primary care and complementary medicine, shows many valuable ways for CAM research. Without questioning the importance of clinical studies and the adaption of biomedical research methods to CAM, this supplement shows the need for new ways in CAM research and for a transfer of knowledge from other fields. One of the lessons to be learnt from PEK is the paradox, that the question about effectiveness of complementary medicine cannot simply be answered through more and more studies on effectiveness! Equally important is a reflection about the reasons, why it is so difficult for CAM research to be acknowledged (as a research field and regarding its results). PEK allows an analysis of equity issues interrelated within an equity circle. This is not only relevant for Switzerland. Anthropological, policy and practice dimensions of equity are identified and linked to different concepts of equity and conceptual frameworks: medical pluralism, cultural imperialism, accountability of reasonableness, distributive justice.

The issues addressed in this supplement are closely connected to two of the four principles of biomedical ethics, i.e. beneficence, non-maleficence, respect for autonomy and justice. So I hope to contribute to acknowledging that respect for autonomy (as closely related to the recognition of medical pluralism), fairness and justice are important issues in research and debate on CAM. Moreover, I hope to show that the dialogue with other fields and disciplines may contribute to sustain the demands for more transparency, democracy and justice in the context of research and health policy.

Florica Marian
Bern

Having been on the review board of PEK and having had first-hand experience of the political processes, the chuzpe and the agenda behind the curtains that led to the decision to stop PEK and to decide against the gist of the data, I welcome this issue which brings together highly pertinent and timely reflections. If we do not start to reflect upon the processes governing research, the agenda behind the driving forces, and the motivations of the main actors, we will never understand outcomes, decisions and science as such. Here, an important starting point is being made. I recommend it warmly to everyone.

Harald Walach
Northampton

KARGER
Fax +49 761 4 52 07 14
E-mail Information@Karger.de
www.karger.com

Accessible online at:
www.karger.com/fok

Dr. rer. med. Florica Marian, lic. phil.
Kollegiale Instanz für Komplementärmedizin KIKOM
Universität Bern, Inselspital Imhoof Pavillon
CH-3010 Bern, Switzerland
Tel. +41 31 6328606, Fax 6324262
E-mail florence.marian@kikom.unibe.ch

Forschende Komplementärmedizin
Wissenschaft · Praxis · Perspektiven

Original Article · Originalarbeit

Forsch Komplementärmed 2007;14(suppl 2):2–9
DOI: 10.1159/000112202

Complementary Medicine: Equity Issues in Evaluation and Policy-Making

Florica Marian

Institute for Complementary Medicine KIKOM, University of Bern, Switzerland

Key Words
Complementary Medicine · Equity · Fairness · Health policy · Evaluation

Summary
The increasing use and practice of complementary and alternative medicine (CAM) all over the world raises important ethical issues for health care providers, researchers and policy-makers. This article addresses the equity issues arising in the context of an evaluation of five complementary therapies provided by general practitioners: homeopathy, anthroposophic medicine, traditional Chinese medicine, neural therapy and phytotherapy. The evaluation was commissioned by the Swiss government in order to provide scientific data to make a policy decision about including these disciplines in basic insurance coverage, if provided by physicians. Both the research process and the related health policy raise a number of equity issues that are explored and further discussed on the basis of Daniels' and Sabin's criteria for fair decision-making as defined in their 'accountability for reasonableness' approach. Combining the lessons learnt from the case study with current approaches to fairness in decision-making and priority-setting, propositions are made in order to increase awareness for transparency and fairness in CAM-related evaluations and policy.

Schlüsselwörter
Komplementärmedizin · Gerechtigkeit · Fairness · Gesundheitspolitik · Evaluation

Zusammenfassung
Das weltweit zunehmende Interesse an Komplementär- und Alternativmedizin (CAM) stellt das Gesundheitssystem und die Gesundheitspolitik vor eine Reihe von Herausforderungen und ethischen Fragen. Im Rahmen des nationalen Forschungsprojekts PEK (Programm Evaluation Komplementärmedizin) wurden 5 Disziplinen bezüglich ihrer Wirksamkeit, Zweckmäßigkeit und Wirtschaftlichkeit evaluiert: anthroposophische Medizin, Homöopathie, Neuraltherapie, Phytotherapie und Traditionelle Chinesische Medizin. Diese Evaluation wurde vom Schweizer Bundesrat in Auftrag gegeben, um wissenschaftliche Grundlagen für die Entscheidung über den Verbleib dieser Fachdisziplinen in der Grundversicherung zu liefern. Sowohl der Forschungsprozess als auch der gesundheitspolitische Prozess werfen Fragen nach Gerechtigkeit und Fairness auf, die in diesem Artikel analysiert werden. Verschiedene theoretische Positionen, insbesondere Daniels' und Sabins Kriterien für faire Entscheidungen im Gesundheitswesen, werden im Hinblick auf ihre Relevanz für CAM und den vorgestellten Fall diskutiert. Auf dieser Grundlage werden Vorschläge formuliert für mehr Fairness und Transparenz im Umgang mit CAM im Rahmen von Evaluationen und Gesundheitspolitik.

Introduction and Background

Complementary medicine can be defined as 'diagnosis, treatment and/or prevention which complements mainstream medicine by contribution to a common whole, by satisfying a demand not met by orthodoxy or by diversifying the conceptual frameworks of medicine' [1]. The increasing use of complementary medicine has led to a growing debate and research activity including scientific, political, legal and ethical issues. The current literature about ethical issues concerning comple-

KARGER

Fax +49 761 4 52 07 14
E-mail Information@Karger.de
www.karger.com

Accessible online at:
www.karger.com/fok

Dr. rer. med. Florica Marian, lic. phil.
Kollegiale Instanz für Komplementärmedizin KIKOM
Universität Bern, Inselspital Imhoof Pavillon
CH-3010 Bern, Switzerland
Tel. +41 31 6328606, Fax 6324262
E-mail florence.marian@kikom.unibe.ch

mentary medicine covers a broad range of topics such as its legal status, informed consent, obligations of conventional physicians regarding complementary medicine, research issues and safety [2–5]. Less attention has been devoted to equity issues concerning research and politics in the field of complementary and alternative medicine (CAM).

In Switzerland, the former Minister of Health, Ruth Dreifuss, had decided to admit on a provisional basis until 2005 five CAM therapies provided by physicians to the compulsory health insurance coverage: homeopathy, anthroposophic medicine, neural therapy, phytotherapy and traditional Chinese medicine (TCM). A nationwide evaluation of these disciplines was then commissioned by the government to assess their effectiveness, suitability and cost-effectiveness in order to provide a scientific basis for deciding whether these methods should be retained under basic health coverage. To this end, from 1998 to December 2005 the Complementary Medicine Evaluation Programme (Programm Evaluation Komplementärmedizin – PEK) was carried out and financed with approximately 7 million SFR (12 million EUR) from public sources. In that time, the government as well as the responsible authorities for the project changed, which had important implications on the research and decision-making process. In June 2005, i.e. before the results of PEK had been finally evaluated, published and discussed, the Minister of Health and Home Affairs, Pascal Couchepin, decided to withdraw the 5 methods in question from basic health coverage.

In this article, I will first provide an overview of the equity issues arising within PEK. These will be further discussed in the context of Daniels' and Sabin's framework of accountability for reasonableness (A4R) [6] including its recent developments. Finally, I will propose a framework aimed at increasing awareness for equity and fairness in policy issues related to complementary medicine.

Equity Issues in the Programme for the Evaluation of Complementary Medicine

Both research and health policy aspects of PEK have been described and analyzed in several articles and reports: evaluation of the PEK process [Hess, unpublished], policy analysis [8], documents written by members of the PEK Steering Committee and Review Board [9–13]. In these documents, equity and fairness issues are mentioned or implicitly addressed with respect to (1) the evaluation concept, (2) the research and decision-making process, and (3) the consequences of the health policy decision.

Evaluation Concept

The evaluation concept of PEK was the result of a broad consensus process which included representatives of complementary medicine, conventional medicine, methodologists and policy-makers. An international review board oversaw the project. PEK comprised two elements: empirical studies conducted in Swiss primary care, and reviews of the literature.

The first element consisted of observational studies assessing the prevalence of therapies, profiles of providers and users, diagnostic and therapeutic procedures used by physicians, and perceived effectiveness and satisfaction in patients [14]. These studies included physicians belonging to the medical associations of the 5 disciplines in question and their patients. The comparison was made with a representative sample of physicians practising conventional medicine and their patients [15–17]. Clinical studies aiming to prospectively compare the effects of the target therapies with those of conventional therapies on selected syndromes were blocked by the local ethical committee. This was possibly due to a combination of two factors: an existing bias against CAM in the ethics committee and a lack of agreement about the methodological quality of the planned studies.

The second element of PEK systematically compiled and reviewed the internationally available literature on efficacy, appropriateness and cost-effectiveness [18, 19]. These studies were carried out by research institutes affiliated to several universities [14].

Research and Decision-Making Process

From 1998 to 2004, the main steps in the design and the realization of the studies were the results of a sometimes difficult but always fair, constructive and transparent consensus process between representatives of the research institutes, methodologists, experts for conventional and complementary disciplines and policy-makers. Accordingly, PEK was described as a fair attempt of an organized dialogue between conventional and complementary medicine [13].

After 5 years of research and after changes had taken place at the political level, responsibility for the project was transferred to the Swiss Federal Office of Public Health (FOPH). In 2004, the FOPH was informed about the initial results, which were favourable to CAM methods. The FOPH reaction, however, aimed to prohibit publication of these results. To this end, the authorities took legally correct but democratically problematic administrative steps such as not allowing researchers to present or publish the results, not allowing collaborating experts access to data and firing scientific collaborators that worked on PEK publications. Even the international review board was prevented from commenting on the draft and the final report before the decision was made; and the final report together with a dossier that protested the procedures was only released after firm protest from the review board [10, 11]. Finally, in June 2005 the Federal Council decided to exclude the 5 CAM disciplines in question from compulsory health coverage. Although some serious limitations of the PEK studies have to be acknowledged (such as the low answer rate of

physicians), their results indicate a favourable assessment with regard to patient satisfaction and safety, as well as some, although limited, positive evidence for cost-effectiveness [14].
A striking example of perceived lack of fairness concerns the interpretation of evidence and the justification of the decision. For instance, the lack of randomised controlled trials (RCT) in the field was interpreted by the authorities as a lack of evidence, whereas evidence from the PEK surveys that was in favour of CAM, i.e. patient satisfaction, perceived effectiveness, safety and costs, was ignored by the policy-makers, who called any scientific data 'waste products which do not bear any relevance to the political decision' [9]. Furthermore, the necessity to reduce health care expenditures was used as an argument to justify the policy decision. This argument, however, is not supported by data. The provisional inclusion of the 5 disciplines in basic insurance was neither a relevant cost factor, nor will their exclusion save significant costs [8]. According to the final report, the total cost impact of complementary medicine is quite low, and cost-effectiveness of 2 of the disciplines assessed, namely anthroposophic medicine and homeopathy, is even positive [14]. Third, there is reason to assume that excluding complementary medicine from basic health coverage will not save costs. In fact, even the opposite may happen and malpractice be encouraged: As in the current reimbursement scheme (Tarmed) it is not obligatory to declare the kind of diagnostic or therapeutic procedure practised, services specific to complementary medicine, if provided by physicians, can be charged as conventional medicine and thus be reimbursed, possibly at a higher cost.
It is important to point this out, since the argumentation of the authorities as well as information in the media 'seem to imply that the Swiss decision was based on evidence about the higher costs and ineffectiveness of complementary medicine. Very likely, the opposite was true: the data probably suggested some cost-effectiveness, and they certainly did not imply zero effectiveness. But this information was held back from the public in order to veil the political nature of the decision' [9].
Furthermore, the official justification of the decision mentions additional analyses of the PEK data on which the decision was based as well, but does not give any details of the methodology, results and references regarding these analyses [10], while the data themselves were barred from public or scientific scrutiny.

Impact and Consequences of the Health Policy

The impact and the consequences of the political decision are more complex and controversial than the issues mentioned above. Nevertheless, some consequences may be expected on access to care, quality of care, medical education and research funding.
With respect to the equity of the Swiss health care system, Crivelli assumes that the PEK policy will have neither a negative nor a positive impact on general equity and access to care, which will still be very good as compared to other countries [8]. An important part of the services, that were explicitly reimbursed as complementary medicine during the 5 years of the PEK evaluation, can still be reimbursed in the future, though in a disguised way, namely as services that belong to conventional medicine. Even if this overall appreciation of the equity of the system may be correct, it remains an issue of concern. First, even if in daily practice insurers are bound by law to accept everybody into basic health coverage, coverage of an additional insurance may be subject to the respective health status. As patients who seek complementary medicine tend to be more chronically and more severely ill, they will be discriminated if CAM is not included in the compulsory coverage [17]. This leads to a discrimination against low-income patients as well as against chronically ill and elderly patients who suffer from multiple conditions. Furthermore, patients who suffer from conditions for which effective complementary but no conventional treatments exist (so-called 'effectiveness gaps' [20]) may also be discriminated against. Coverage limitations may also have a negative impact upon information about and access to care, because therapies that are not reimbursed tend to be prescribed less [21].
The attitude and the behaviour of the authorities as well as 'the signal effect' [8] of their decision may affect opinions, attitudes, motivations and behaviours of patients and physicians in several ways. Patients may be dissuaded from seeking complementary care or discussing CAM treatment options with their physicians, who may also be less motivated to inform themselves about CAM treatment options and to acquire further qualifications to practise CAM [22]. The ethical issues addressed here, namely that physicians have a duty to inform themselves and their patients about CAM options, have been addressed in the USA, but are still neglected in Europe [3, 23, 24]. During the evaluation period, the inclusion of the 5 CAM disciplines in basic insurance coverage was linked to an additional qualification recognized and certified by the FMH (Foederatio Medicorum Helvetica – Association of Swiss Physicians). This qualification may be less important and less attractive in the future, with corresponding consequences on the quality of CAM practice, if physicians may declare diagnostic and therapeutic procedures of CAM as conventional medicine. It is also uncertain to what extent this qualification will be recognized and certified by the FMH in the future.
Given the complexity and interconnectedness of the issues addressed, several 'systemic' effects have to be expected on access to and quality of care, on medical education and research funding, in the short-, middle- and long-term, but they are difficult to predict.

Equity Issues in PEK: Issues of Distributive Justice?

In the case of PEK, the structures, the organisation as well as the evaluation model were perceived as fair with respect to

Table 1. Equity issues in PEK: Overview of perceived aspects

Aspects of equity	Arising in PEK
Personal use with respect to	
Persons or group of persons	Political authorities after 2004
Their activities and behaviours	Strategy of the authorities during research and decision-making process
Their value judgements, assessments, estimations	Negative opinion about CAM and political nature of the decision
Institutional use	
Procedures, rules and laws	Lack of transparency in decision-making Deviation from conventional standards (lack of review process, lack of transparency) Academic rules as obstacle to CAM research
Social and political institutions	Sponsoring bias and conflict of interest
Theoretical use	
Statements, theories, principles, models	Normative bias expressed in the justification of the decision and statements to the media
Procedural use	
Distributive procedures	Lack of similar evaluations of conventional therapies included in basic health coverage
Consequences	
Reciprocity of exchanges	Relationship between engagement of involved stakeholders and results of process
Results of procedures	Consequences on access to care, quality of care, medical education, research funding, 'systemic impact'
Distribution of natural or historical goods	Non-recognition of CAM within mainstream medicine

(1) the distribution of tasks and responsibilities between representatives of conventional and complementary medicine, and (2) the evaluation model, as resulting from a broad consensus between the different stakeholders, and taking into account the specificity of the health technologies assessed. On the other hand, several stakeholders perceived the authorities' attitude after the changes in the political responsibility for the project, the decision-making process, the decision itself as well as their consequences as lacking fairness and as discriminating against complementary medicine. In the meantime, awareness of some equity-related concerns has extended to several politicians who have requested an official audit of the process. Further equity issues related to the sponsoring of the studies and to academic rules were observed by the author as a senior researcher involved in the PEK studies [17]. The phenomenon of sponsorship bias in bio-medical research is well known and has been described on various occasions [25–27]. PEK has shown that public funding, as well, may lead to bias and misuse of power. Two questions have arisen after the change of authorities in 2004. (1) How is it possible that actions such as prohibiting researchers from presenting and publishing results are taken in a democratic country? (2) Why did researchers accept such a strategy without protest?

One possible explanation for these incidents may be the power of the Swiss Federal Office of Public Health (FOPH) as the owner of the PEK data and at the same time a major sponsor for other health care related research. Criticising PEK-related undemocratic actions of the FOPH would have jeopardized current and future sponsoring as well as further collaboration between researchers and the FOPH. A personal anecdote may illustrate the arbitrariness typical for daily routine during the PEK after the change of leading authorities in 2004: Only in the very last minute, the FOPH prohibited researchers from presenting PEK results in a conference organized at the University of Bern on 21 April 2005 [11]. As a consequence, the author was threatened with dismissal even if she only attended the conference as a participant. On the same day, a colleague from the same institute, yet not involved in PEK, was sent to that conference and asked to record on tape all contributions. Given the power of the FOPH as the owner of the data, protests would have made impossible further work on PEK data and would thus have supported the FOPH strategy as described above. Conflicts of interest, sponsorship and publication bias are well known and have been repeatedly described in bio-medical and pharmaceutical research [25]. PEK has shown that they may also occur in the case of public funding, even if the funding institution by contract is not to be involved in data analysis and publication.

Another equity issue is related to the academic rules in the German speaking part of Switzerland, in which an academic post-doctoral qualification (habilitation) is a prerequisite for supervising PhD students. Although there is a chair for complementary medicine (divided among 4 CAM disciplines) at the University of Bern, the Chair holders (4 lecturers) cannot automatically supervise medical dissertations autonomously, but need support from their colleagues. This situation of dependence arising from co-directorates may be associated with misuse of power and arbitrariness. The difficulty to publish PEK-related data after the political decision was made is also linked with an institutional situation discriminating against CAM. The latter was also visible in the negative decision of the Ethical Committee of the Canton of Bern against further prospective studies on CAM therapies within PEK, based on the ground that they were not conceived as randomised studies. This hidden power of ethical committees is another issue worthy of consideration in the context of equity issues.

The broad range of situations in which equity issues implicitly or explicitly arose within PEK is shown in table 1. This overview was first developed by Horn and Scarano [28] and aimed at giving an overview of situations in which equity issues may have to be addressed.

Upon reflecting PEK-related equity issues, questions arise about the definition of equity, the objectivity of statements as well as the lack of fairness in process and decision-making. It is well known that a lack of equity is much more evident and much easier to feel, notice and describe than to define what equity and fairness in fact are [29]. It is also difficult to bridge the gap between the practical world of policy and theoretical discussions [30]. Equity issues in the context of CAM have not yet been analyzed, neither with respect to theory nor with respect to practice. The following is an attempt to link some definitions and reflections about equity, justice and fairness with PEK and CAM. 'Equity means social justice or fairness; it is an ethical concept, grounded in principles of distributive justice' [31]. According to Spaemann, justice is the recognition of a fundamental symmetry in the relationships between persons, especially with respect to the distribution of limited resources. This symmetry does not mean absolute equality, but asymmetry has to be explained and justified. The justification must be done such that fair-minded persons can agree with this asymmetry. If a person is subject to discriminating measures that are not or cannot be justified, the fundamental symmetry is violated. Justice does not imply that everyone shall have the same. It implies that criteria for the distribution of burden and compensations should not be biased. Therefore, Justitia, the iconic representation of justice, is represented as blindfold: justice means impartiality [32]. Principles fostering impartiality are a common good in humankind, as an Egyptian rule (1500 B.C.) shows: 'Consider someone you know the same as anyone you do not know, and someone who is near to you the same as anyone whose house is far' [33]. In the case of PEK, one condition for a fair process would have been impartiality of the authorities, as it could be observed before the political change in 2004. Impartiality as a basic value and attitude would have probably ensured fair procedures. Given the debate and controversy about the effectiveness of CAM in general and about the limitations of the PEK studies, impartiality with respect to the decision itself would have been extremely difficult to achieve. Nevertheless, impartiality could have been strived for during the decision-making process by balancing pros and cons, by making that process transparent, by involving the stakeholders and by respecting standards regarding the review of the final PEK report [10]. Justice is symbolized by a balance, representing the duty to balance and distribute adequately. The distinction between distributive justice and corrective justice was first described by Aristotle and further developed in the Middle Ages by scholastic philosophers such as Thomas Aquinas (justitia distributiva and justitia commutativa or correctiva) [28]. The concept of distributive justice implies the distribution of material and non-material goods such as honours and duties according to the principle of geometrical proportionality [34]. The perceived lack of fairness in the PEK is implicitly based on this concept. Accordingly, there is no reason to discriminate against physicians who provide complementary medicine, nor against their patients, nor against researchers in that field and to treat them with less respect than if any other field would be concerned. The concept of corrective justice (in German 'ausgleichende Gerechtigkeit') is based on arithmetical equality and the principle of reciprocity, also relevant in the context of PEK. Recent discussions about evidence-based health policy emphasize the importance of context, which includes all factors that influence the environment in which a decision is made and applied [35]. Such factors include the distribution of research funding, recognition, academic representation, none of which is proportional to CAM use. Furthermore, in the case of PEK, providers of complementary medicine are de facto practising an integrative medical approach and are at least equally qualified as their conventional colleagues. Balancing such national and international context factors would have contributed to compensate (ausgleichen) existing discrimination against CAM.

Criteria for Fairness in Decision-Making: Accountability for Reasonableness

A key problem associated both with the case of PEK and with priority-setting in general is fairness of a decision. This is the main question addressed in the A4R framework in the context of US managed care [6]. According to that framework, a decision in health care may be considered as fair if it ensures that four conditions are satisfied.

1. Publicity: Decisions and their rationales must be publicly accessible.
2. Relevance: These rationales must rest on information and principled arguments that fair-minded parties (people predisposed to working together under rules of mutual cooperation) can agree are relevant to deciding how to meet the diverse needs of a population under necessary resource constraints.
3. Appeals: There is a mechanism for challenging and disputing decisions on priorities, including the opportunity to revise decisions in the light of further evidence or arguments.

Table 2. Considerations for fairness in CAM research and policy

Equity issue	Considerations
Evaluation concept	Integrate a broad range of evidence. Include quantitative and qualitative evaluation models. Accept the plurality of medical systems and evaluation models. Make value judgements explicit.
Research funding	Transparency about sponsor-driven control over data and results. Transparency about conflicts of interest. Amount of public funding proportional to CAM use in the population.
Research process	Ensure that all stakeholders (including patients) are represented at all stages of the research process. Take ethical issues into account. Apply A4R conditions: publicity, relevance, appeal, enforcement and empowerment.
Health policy and decision-making	Apply A4R conditions: publicity, relevance, appeal, enforcement and empowerment. Make value judgements explicit.
Priority-setting	Avoid discrimination of patients on the basis of income and burden of disease. Reflect consequences on equity issues. Reflect consequences of patient and provider autonomy.
Public debate	Public debate about the role of ideology in health policy decisions.
Process evaluation	Examine if stakeholders – felt understood and engaged – consider decision justified and reasonable – felt fairly treated

4. Enforcement: There is either voluntary or public regulation of the process in order to ensure that conditions 1 through 3 are met.

Although developed in the empirical context of US managed care, the strength of A4R is ethically rooted in theories of democratic deliberation, philosophical ethics and political philosophy. These roots connect the process of priority-setting in health care with broader democratic processes. A4R has been widely discussed and developed further. Observing that power differences in the decision-making context may be a serious impediment for the fairness of the process, Gibson and colleagues have proposed to add the condition of 'empowerment' to the A4R framework [36]. Power differences exist when 'some individuals and groups are better positioned than others to influence priority-setting outcomes. If the interests of some individuals or groups are allowed to dominate the context within which priority setting decisions are made, then the outcomes of priority setting may fail to be fair' [36]. This is exactly what occurred in the case of PEK, i.e. the problem of power was acknowledged to be a central one [11]. Consequently, the 'empowerment condition' states that efforts should be made to minimize power differences in the decision-making context and to optimize effective opportunities for participation [36]. Empowerment in terms of an integration of stakeholder perspectives is also an issue of concern in PEK, although it has not yet been addressed in the articles about PEK. Neither patient representatives nor ethicists were represented and involved at any stage of the process, which contradicts theory, and increasingly also practice, of Health Technology Assessments. Therefore, it would be worth to consider the following questions developed in the context of priority-setting and decision-making [37]:

- Did stakeholders and decision-makers consider the priority-setting process worth their while?
- Did the stakeholders feel understood and engaged in the priority-setting process?
- Did the stakeholders consider the decision-making process and the decision justified and reasonable?
- Did both 'winners' and 'losers' feel that they had been fairly treated?

This short introduction to the A4R approach may demonstrate that it should be acknowledged and taken into account in CAM-related discussions [38]. It is worth noticing that the A4R approach has been described before in a report about priority-setting in the Swiss health system [39]. As weaknesses of the Swiss health care system that report identifies a lack of transparency and stakeholders' involvement in health policy decisions [39].

Considerations for Fairness in CAM Research and Policy

On the basis of the critical analysis of PEK and the reflections about lessons to be learned, a framework has been developed to integrate CAM-related issues with the A4R approach and its current developments [6, 36, 37, 40] (table 2).

Concluding Remarks

A broad range of equity issues that arose in PEK was described in this article and linked to concepts of justice and fairness, especially to the A4R approach of Daniels and Sabin. Having integrated lessons from PEK with these theoretical approaches, propositions were made how to increase fairness in CAM-related evaluations and policy-making. Reflection on PEK in the light of current discussions in related fields shows that some issues of concern have also been described in other fields. For example, the fact that research tends to play a neglected role in health policy decisions mostly driven by ideology and other values [41–43]. Nevertheless, we would not have expected such behaviour of the authorities, for PEK was created to support and inform a policy decision. Increasing awareness that in priority-setting simple solutions are not appropriate to the complexity of modern health care systems has led to an international trend towards more transparency, integration of a broad range of evidence, integration of stakeholder perspectives and context factors in decision-making [35, 7]. PEK-related policy-making, however, reveals the opposite.

This article is a first attempt to link actual discussions about fairness in decision-making and theoretical considerations about equity to the field of CAM. Given the plurality of equity issues and the complexity of the interdisciplinary issues arising, this is a field that should be further explored in future research. Three approaches were combined in this article:

- an empirical approach (based on articles and reports of stakeholders),
- a normative approach (reflections about what a fair process would look like),
- a theoretical approach (linking equity concepts to the field of CAM)

An important limitation of this article is that most of the articles and reports that document equity issues are written by researchers or stakeholders involved in CAM and/or CAM research. Taking this limitation into account, the conceptual frameworks presented in this article as well as current developments and discussion in the respective fields offer valuable approaches to CAM-related decision-making. If applied to the context of complementary medicine, these approaches may sustain the claim for more democracy and justice, more transparency and involvement of stakeholders in research and decision-making processes.

Acknowledgements

This study was supported by the Merkur-Rafael Foundation, the Fondation Homéopathique Pierre Schmidt and the University of Bern. I thank Klaus von Ammon, Bryn William-Jones, Johan Hulson, Peter Heusser and Pedro Koch for their comments on an earlier version of this paper. I thank Harald Walach for the review of this manuscript.

Literatur

1 Ernst E, Cohen MH, Stone J: Ethical problems arising in evidence based complementary and alternative medicine. J Med Ethics 2004;30:156–159.
2 Miller FG, Emanuel EJ, Rosenstein DL, Straus SE: Ethical issues concerning research in complementary and alternative medicine. Jama 2004;291: 599–604.
3 Sugarman J, Burk L: Physicians' ethical obligations regarding alternative medicine. Jama 1998;280: 1623–1625.
4 Adams KE, Cohen MH, Eisenberg D, Jonsen AR: Ethical considerations of complementary and alternative medical therapies in conventional medical settings. Ann Intern Med 2002;137:660–664.
5 Kerridge IH, McPhee JR: Ethical and legal issues at the interface of complementary and conventional medicine. Med J Aust 2004;181:164–166.
6 Daniels N, Sabin J: The ethics of accountability in managed care reform. Health Aff (Millwood) 1998; 17:50–64.
7 Slowther A, Ford S, Schofield T: Ethics of evidence based medicine in the primary care setting. J Med Ethics 2004;30:151–155.
8 Crivelli L: Slimming diet for the FHIA benefit basket; in: Health Policy Monitor. Lugano, Universita della Svizzera Italiana, 2005.
9 Walach H: The Swiss program for the evaluation of complementary medicine (PEK). J Altern Complement Med 2006;12:231–232.
10 Walach H, Linde K, Eichenberger R, Stalder H, Borlum Kristensen F, Kleijnen J: Summary consensus statement of the Review Board of the Swiss Complementary Medicine Evaluation Programme, (Programm Evaluation Komplementärmedizin, PEK) regarding the PEK process and products. Homeopathy 2006;95:28–30.
11 Heusser P: Medizin und Macht am Beispiel des Programms Evaluation Komplementärmedizin PEK; in Ausfeld-Hafter B (ed): Medizin und Macht. Die Arzt-Patienten-Beziehung im Wandel: Mehr Entscheidungsfreiheit? Bern, Peter Lang, 2007.
12 Heusser P: PEK und BAG: Probleme beim Programm Evaluation Komplementärmedizin. Schweiz Ärzteztg 2006;87:899–903.
13 Melchart D: Das Programm zur Evaluation der Komplementärmedizin (PEK) – ein fairer Versuch eines organisierten Dialogs zwischen Schulmedizin und Komplementärmedizin. Schweiz Ärzteztg 2005;86:934–937.
14 Melchart D, Mitscherlich F, Amiet M, Eichenberger R, Koch P: Programm Evaluation Komplementärmedizin (PEK) Schlussbericht. Bern, Bundesamt für Gesundheit, 2005.
15 Busato A, Donges A, Herren S, Widmer M, Marian F: Health status and health care utilisation of patients in complementary and conventional primary care in Switzerland – an observational study. Fam Pract 2006;23:116–124.
16 Widmer M, Herren S, Donges A, Marian F, Busato A: Complementary and conventional medicine in Switzerland: Comparing characteristics of general practitioners. Forsch Komplementärmed 2006;13: 234–240.
17 Marian F, Widmer M, Herren S, Donges A, Busato A: Physicians' philosophy of care: a comparison of complementary and conventional medicine. Forsch Komplementärmed 2006;13:70–77.
18 Walach H, Heusser P: [Effective or not? The decision is yours! – the PEK HTA reports]. Forsch Komplementärmed 2006;13(suppl 2):2–3.
19 Nartey L, Huwiler-Muntener K, Shang A, Liewald K, Juni P, Egger M: Matched-pair study showed higher quality of placebo-controlled trials in Western phytotherapy than conventional medicine. J Clin Epidemiol 2007;60:787–794.

20 Shang A, Huwiler K, Nartey L, Juni P, Egger M: Placebo-controlled trials of Chinese herbal medicine and conventional medicine – comparative study. Int J Epidemiol 2007;36:1086–1092.
21 Shang A, Huwiler-Muntener K, Nartey L, Juni P, Dorig S, Sterne JA, Pewsner D, Egger M: Are the clinical effects of homoeopathy placebo effects? Comparative study of placebo-controlled trials of homoeopathy and allopathy. Lancet 2005;366: 726–732.
22 Fisher P, van Haselen R, Hardy K, Berkovitz S, McCarney R: Effectiveness gaps: a new concept for evaluating health service and research needs applied to complementary and alternative medicine. J Altern Complement Med 2004;10:627–632.
23 Wynia MK, VanGeest JB, Cummins DS, Wilson IB: Do physicians not offer useful services because of coverage restrictions? Health Aff (Millwood) 2003; 22:190–197.
24 Lemann D: Komplementärmedizin und Krankenkassen. Wie rechnen komplementärmedizinisch tätige Ärzte zukünftig mit den Krankenkassen ab? Schweiz Z Ganzheitsmed 2005:266–268.
25 Brophy E: Does a doctor have a duty to provide information and advice about complementary and alternative medicine? J Law Med 2003;10:271–284.
26 Sugarman J: Informed consent, shared decision-making, and complementary and alternative medicine. J Law Med Ethics 2003;31:247–250.
27 Gotzsche PC: Research integrity and pharmaceutical industry sponsorship. Trial registration, transparency and less reliance on industry trials are essential. Med J Aust 2005;182:549–550.
28 Abraham J: The pharmaceutical industry as a political player. Lancet 2002;360:1498–1502.
29 Abraham J: Transnational industrial power, the medical profession and the regulatory state: adverse drug reactions and the crisis over the safety of Halcion in the Netherlands and the UK. Soc Sci Med 2002;55:1671–1690.
30 Horn C, Scarano N (eds): Philosophie der Gerechtigkeit. Texte der Antike bis zur Gegenwart. Frankfurt/M., Suhrkamp, 2002.
31 Laupies F: La justice. Premières leçons. Paris, Presses Universitaires de France, 2005.
32 Culyer AJ: Equity – some theory and its policy implications. J Med Ethics 2001;27:275–283.
33 Braveman P, Gruskin S: Defining equity in health. J Epidemiol Community Health 2003;57:254–258.
34 Schweppenhäuser G: Grundbegriffe der Ethik. Hamburg, Junius, 2003.
35 Höffe O: Gerechtigkeit. Eine philosophische Einführung. München, Beck, 2004.
36 Aristoteles: Nikomachische Ethik. Stuttgart, Reclam, 1969.
37 Dobrow MJ, Goel V, Upshur RE: Evidence-based health policy: context and utilisation. Soc Sci Med 2004;58:207–217.
38 Gibson JL, Martin DK, Singer PA: Priority setting in hospitals: fairness, inclusiveness, and the problem of institutional power differences. Soc Sci Med 2005;61:2355–2362.
39 Gibson JL, Martin DK, Singer PA: Setting priorities in health care organizations: criteria, processes, and parameters of success. BMC Health Serv Res 2004;4:25.
40 Peacock S, Ruta D, Mitton C, Donaldson C, Bate A, Murtagh M: Using economics to set pragmatic and ethical priorities. BMJ 2006;332:482–485.
41 Mittelverteilung im schweizerischen Gesundheitswesen. Zusammenfassung der Befunde und Empfehlungen; in Schopper D, Baumann-Hölzle R, Tanner M (eds): Schweizerisches Tropeninstitut, Dialog Ethik, 2001.
42 Gibson JL, Martin DK, Singer PA: Priority setting for new technologies in medicine: a transdisciplinary study. BMC Health Serv Res 2002;2:14.
43 Black N: Evidence based policy: proceed with care. BMJ 2001;323:275–279.

Forschende Komplementärmedizin
Wissenschaft • Praxis • Perspektiven

Essay

Forsch Komplementärmed 2007;14(suppl 2):10–18
DOI: 10.1159/000112319

Medical Pluralism: Global Perspectives on Equity Issues

Florica Marian

Institute for Complementary Medicine KIKOM, University of Bern, Switzerland

Key Words
Medical Pluralism · Complementary Medicine · Traditional Medicine · Equity · Fairness

Summary
Over the last decades, awareness has increased about the phenomenon of medical pluralism and the importance to integrate biomedicine and other forms of health care. The broad variety of healing cultures existing alongside biomedicine is called complementary or alternative medicine (CAM) in industrialized countries and traditional medicine (TM) in developing countries. Considerable debate has arisen about ethical problems related to the growing use of CAM in industrialized countries. This article focuses on equity issues and aims to consider them from a global perspective of medical pluralism. Several dimensions of equity are explored and their interrelatedness discussed: access to care, research (paradigm and founding) and recognition. This so-called 'equity circle' is then related to Iris Marion Young's justice theory and particularly to the concepts of cultural imperialism, powerlessness and marginalisation.

Schlüsselwörter
Pluralismus in der Medizin · Komplementärmedizin · Traditionelle Medizin · Gerechtigkeit · Fairness

Zusammenfassung
In den letzten Jahrzehnten hat das Bewusstsein für Pluralismus in der Medizin und für die Notwendigkeit, verschiedene medizinische Ansätze im Gesundheitswesen zu integrieren, zugenommen. Die große Vielfalt an therapeutischen Ansätzen und medizinischen Systemen, die neben oder ergänzend zur Biomedizin existieren, ist als Komplementär- und Alternativmedizin (CAM) oder auch als Traditionelle Medizin (TM) bekannt. Das wachsende Interesse an CAM in Industrieländern sowie an TM in Entwicklungsländern ist mit einer Reihe ethischer Fragestellungen und Herausforderungen verbunden, welche in den letzten Jahren zunehmend erforscht wurden. Eine Ausnahme bilden die Fragen nach Gerechtigkeit und Fairness. Diese haben im Zusammenhang mit CAM und TM bisher wenig Beachtung gefunden. In diesem Artikel werden einige zusammengehörende Dimensionen und Aspekte von Gerechtigkeit und Fairness im Kontext von CAM/TM analysiert: Zugang zur Versorgung, Forschung (Paradigma und Finanzierung), Anerkennung. Anhand von Iris Marion Youngs Konzept des Kulturimperialismus werden weiterführende Aspekte zum Verständnis der Fragen von Gerechtigkeit im CAM-Kontext aufgezeigt.

Introduction

We can observe the phenomena of medical pluralism and the use of different forms of health care all over the world. These include biomedicine as well as a multitude of medical and therapeutic healing cultures, which are commonly defined as complementary, alternative (CAM) or non-conventional medicine in industrialized countries and as traditional medicine (TM) in developing countries. According to the WHO, both CAM and TM refer to health practices, approaches, knowl-

KARGER
Fax +49 761 4 52 07 14
E-mail Information@Karger.de
www.karger.com

Accessible online at:
www.karger.com/fok

Dr. rer. med. Florica Marian, lic. phil.
Kollegiale Instanz für Komplementärmedizin KIKOM
Universität Bern, Inselspital Imhoof Pavillon
CH-3010 Bern, Switzerland
Tel. +41 31 6328606, Fax 6324262
E-mail florence.marian@kikom.unibe.ch

edge and beliefs comprising plant, animal, and mineral-based medicines, spiritual therapies, manual techniques and exercises, applied singularly or in combination to treat, diagnose, and prevent illness or maintain well-being [1, 2]. The increasing use of CAM/TM is associated with several ethical issues examined in current research. These include general issues [3–5], legal issues [4, 6–9], research ethics [10, 11], decision-making and informed consent [12–16]. Due to the large number and variety of types, definitions and legal status of TM/CAM, research on equity issues has been neglected to date. The aim of this article is to lay out some equity issues that arise from the increasing use of TM/CAM from the global perspective of medical pluralism.

This article is structured as follows: after briefly introducing medical pluralism, I will explore equity issues such as access to care, research (paradigm and funding) and recognition. After demonstrating their interrelatedness within an equity circle, an attempt will be made in the third section to grasp some essential dimensions of justice in the context of CAM on the basis of Iris Marion Young's theory of justice.

Context of Medical Pluralism

Pluralism is basically legitimized through core principles of social and political justice: the right to freedom and free choice [17]. In this context, it is closely related to respect for autonomy as one of the four principles of medical ethics (the other principles being beneficience, non-maleficience and justice) [18]. According to Beauchamp and Childress [18], respect for autonomy implies 'to acknowledge that person's right to hold views, to make choices, and to take actions based on personal values and beliefs'. Respect for autonomy is mostly understood as a patient's right to choose his therapy, but it also implies the therapeutic freedom of health care providers in general [19]. The increasing importance of the autonomy principle is associated with broad societal changes concerning goals of medicine and health care and with paradigmatic changes such as the transition from a biomedical to a more patient-centred paradigm [20]. Thus, recognizing medical pluralism means acknowledging these changes. Moreover, recognizing medical pluralism has been acknowledged as central issue towards fairness and understanding of CAM therapies as well as one of five major ethical commitments that must be embraced in the context of an ethical framework for CAM research, practice and policy [21]. Claims for the recognition of medical pluralism are based on the argument that many CAM therapies partly or fully originate from healing systems and traditions other than biomedicine. Thus, any investigation or evaluation of CAM therapies should include a moral commitment to openness regarding the meaning of health and healing and regarding innovative ways of increasing evidence and knowledge [21]. Medical pluralism as a value and commitment requires 'suspending any categorial disbelief in CAM therapies' and an attitude of 'skepticism about any claim that conventional biomedical research and practice exhaustively account for the human experience of health and healing, combined with diligent efforts to discern the significance, safety and efficacy of CAM therapies' [21]. Accordingly, official recognition, promotion and integration of CAM into all areas of health care systems is part of the WHO strategy [1, 2]. Empirical data published in WHO documents sustain these claims [1, 2]. In China, traditional herbal preparations account for 30–50% of the total medical consumption In Africa, up to 80% of the population uses traditional medicine for primary health care. In Ghana, Mali, Nigeria and Zambia, 60% of children with high fever resulting from malaria are treated with herbal medicines in the first instance. In Taiwan, 60% of the population use different healing systems including biomedicine.

In Europe, North America and other industrialized regions, more than 50% of the population have used CAM at least once. In Germany, 90% of the population have used a natural remedy at some point in their life. Between 1995 and 2000, the number of doctors licensed in natural medicine almost doubled. In the United States, 158 million of the adult population use complementary medicines and 17 billion USD were spent on traditional remedies in 2000. Surveys from industrialized countries indicate that 35–50% of the population use some form of complementary therapies [1, 2, 22, 23]. Recognition of pluralism is also an implicit or explicit issue in the ongoing discussions about the different ways of co-existence of different forms of health care within one and the same health care system. Some Asian countries such as China, South Korea and India have incorporated traditional health systems into their national health policies. In the United States and Europe, a considerable body of the literature argues for integrating conventional and complementary medicine in the health care system and offers patients the 'best of both worlds' [24–26].

Finally, pluralism has been seen as an ethical model that promotes cooperation and respect between different therapeutic approaches, while at the same time it preserves their integrity [27]. In summary, the different aspects giving a framework for the discussion of ethical and equity issues are:

- pluralism as a basic value of democratic societies
- respect for autonomy as a principle of biomedical ethics
- recognition of pluralism as an ethical commitment to CAM practice, policy and research
- pluralism as a model for the co-existence of different healing systems

Considering complementary medicine within the context of medical pluralism implies acknowledging and recognizing different healing systems embedded in their respective culture. Assuming a basic equality between different healing systems is a different starting point to examining equity issues than claiming an overall superiority of the biomedical paradigm and practice. The difficulty is to formulate appropriate questions with respect to equity. As Sen [28] points out, a first step in order to move from the abstract concept of equity to real situations, is to specify 'the space in which equality is to be sought', further asking 'equality of what?', 'equity in what form?'. Equity, in this case is understood as 'a relational concept in which ethical assessments are – at least in part – based on distributional features of one or more variables' [29]. I will first discuss access to care and access to research as two main dimensions in which equity issues in CAM may be explored.

Access to Care

To date, the main equity issue concerning CAM in industrialized countries is access to care. There is little consensus in the literature on what fair access to CAM would signify. Some claim that 'the unequal distribution of CAM within the population violates the fundamental ethical principle of justice' [5], others say 'the benefits of CAM should be freely available to all' [30], or 'patients have fair access to alternative therapies that are known to be safe, effective and appropriate for their conditions' [13]. Different interpretations of the available evidence sustain these claims: '... CAM does more good than harm ...' [5], or '... because little research has evaluated alternative medicine, few data support claims for fair access to these therapies ...' [13]. Access to CAM therapies, obviously, is a matter of justice, but the answer is far from being simple and has to be based on an analysis that considers and balances the four principles of medical ethics, i.e. beneficence, non-maleficence, respect for autonomy and justice. Moreover, access to care and coverage issues should be discussed on the basis of specific CAM definitions relevant in the context of a given national health care system. The mere fact that there is medical pluralism does not necessarily imply a justice issue with regard to public and private assurance funding and coverage of CAM. As health care resources are limited, no health care system is able to cover all services. Therefore, access to CAM therapies has to be negotiated within specific cultural and national contexts. Nevertheless, provision of safe and effective CAM therapies should not depend on a person's income or health status, as is currently the case. This is an issue of concern for both industrialized and developing countries. According to several surveys, common predictors for the use of CAM are higher education and income, chronicity and severity of disease, female gender and a holistic orientation to health. In general, public reimbursement for complementary medicine is not available, and insurance coverage for complementary therapies is either very limited or even completely lacking. Accordingly, in most industrialized countries, CAM is a private and out-of-pocket type of medicine. At the opposite end of the spectrum, more than one third of the population in developing countries have no access to essential medicines (fundamental in basic care, such as antibiotics). Thus, according to the WHO, providing safe and effective TM/CAM therapies could be an important contribution to improve access to health care in those countries [23]. Moreover, patients suffering from conditions for which conventional treatments are not fully effective but for which some evidence for effective complementary treatments exists (so-called 'effectiveness gap' [31]), may find themselves discriminated against in industrialized as well as in developing countries. Yet, due to the increasing recognition of TM, access to care in developing countries seems to be less a problem than qualification of providers. In both industrialized and developing countries, socially or with respect to their health disadvantaged groups have less access to CAM therapies, and this inequity is unnecessary, avoidable, unfair and unjust [32, 33]. Coverage limitations may also have a negative impact on information about and access to care. Accordingly, current research suggests that therapies that are not reimbursed are prescribed three times less [34, 35]. It is reasonable to assume that in the case of CAM these factors operate just as much (if not even more).

Access to CAM therapies is influenced by several factors: information of users and providers, definition of CAM, and acceptance of CAM within a health care system, CAM research, qualification and certification of providers, legislation, coverage and coverage limitations, socio-economic and health status of patients, values of providers and users. Although these issues have specific features depending on the national and continental context, they also have a global dimension and are interconnected within an equity circle.

Access to Research

Lack of evidence of efficacy, efficiency and cost-effectiveness is often associated with CAM, although conventional interventions have at least the same problem to prove their efficacy. There is a broad consensus that there is a need for evidence, and thus research, both in industrialized and developing countries. Yet, the ruling paradigm and funding of research on a dissenting paradigm remain major difficulties.

Paradigm

The dominant research paradigm is based on the biomedical model that defines randomised controlled trials (RCTs) as the highest level of evidence. Limitations of RCTs have been discussed in several contexts such as primary care, health technology assessment and complementary medicine [36–41]. There is increasing consensus that evaluation criteria have to be adapted to the therapy assessed, and that different types of evidence and pluralistic evaluation models have to be considered [9, 36–39]. In practice, however, the dominance of the biomedical paradigm is still discriminating against complementary medicine at several levels. Firstly, as a recent example in Switzerland demonstrates, political decisions concerning complementary medicine tend to support decisions based on RCTs and to ignore bias and limitations inherent in such a model [42–45]. Secondly, some equity issues arising from the

dominance of evidence-based medicine (EBM) described for disadvantaged groups and so-called orphaned fields of medicine may also apply to most of the CAM therapies and the patients using them [46, 47]. With respect to disease burden (chronicity and severity of illness) and gender, the patients using CAM belong to the disadvantaged groups. These groups are underrepresented in decision-making concerning design and methodology as well as participation in the trials, resulting in lack of research corresponding to their needs, of effective therapies, evidence and allocation of resources [46]. Although a considerable amount of research is available for some complementary therapies such as acupuncture or herbal therapy, for the most part of complementary therapies and similarly for orphaned fields of medicine, research evidence is insufficient and financial incentives are lacking to evaluate complex therapeutic interventions by complex conditions [47]. Vos' distinction between 2 ways of reasoning about evidence (the intrusion and the coordination model) is valuable also for CAM [47]. According to the intrusion model, criteria, norms and values of EBM 'intrude' into the worlds of health care providers and patients with possible negative consequences on patient and provider autonomy. Inversely, the coordination model calls for more confidence in the competence of professionals and for more patient participation in all stages of research. Particularly the request to integrate different sources of evidence, such as patient biographic documents and provider knowledge, is also shared by authors in the field of CAM. It is noteworthy that the ethical considerations on EBM from the perspective of disadvantaged groups, orphaned fields and complementary medicine have much in common.
The question if EBM standards are to be adopted in research on complementary medicine is subject to ongoing debates [10, 48, 49].

Research Funding
The question 'Can we trust the evidence in EBM?', summarizes the analysis of some developments in current medical research [45]. Over the last 20 years, commercially sponsored medical research has increased rapidly. According to a recent report of the British House of Lords on the influence of the pharmaceutical industry, 75% of clinical trials published in 'The Lancet', 'The New England Journal of Medicine' and 'The Journal of the American Medical Association' (JAMA) are industry funded [45]. Two thirds thereof are not only sponsored, but also carried out by for-profit research companies whose control over design, data analysis, data interpretation and the publication of results is growing and overtaking that of universities. Recent research suggests that most medical societies receive a large part of their funding from the industry (drug and other medical industries) which also sponsors approximately 70% of physicians' continuing medical education [45].
In summary, driven mostly by commercial factors, current research suggests that many research agendas rather serve the interests of industry than the interests of patients [46, 50]. This tendency in medical research may further accentuate already existing difficulties of CAM research. Firstly, the ties between pharmaceutical industry and medical research and their implications on the level of funding, conducting and publishing research as well as on the level of education are not for the benefit of complementary medicine [50]. Pharmaceutical companies have no interest in sponsoring CAM research, and other public and private funding sources are limited. Yet, the case of the Swiss Programme for the Evaluation of Complementary Medicine (PEK) demonstrates that sponsoring bias may also occur in the case of public funding and if research is carried out in academic institutions. PEK was commissioned by the Swiss Government to evaluate 5 CAM disciplines provided by medical doctors in primary care (anthroposophic medicine, homeopathy, neural therapy and traditional Chinese medicine and phytotherapy) and inform a policy decision. Furthermore, as research tradition in CAM is not well developed, the skills and networks needed to successfully apply for grants from public sources [5] are mostly insufficient. Thus, there is a disparity between the necessity to sustain, support and develop good-quality and evidence-based research in TM/CAM and concrete possibilities to conduct such research [51, 52]. Data from the UK indicate that 10 years ago, only 0.08% of funding for research in the national health system went to complementary medicine [53]. In view of the fact that 25% of the British population used some form of complementary medicine at that time, such a repartitioning of research funding was far from being equitable. In the meantime, although several nationwide CAM research projects have been carried out in Europe, the overall amount of research funding for CAM is still not proportional to the high prevalence of CAM use [54–56].

Equity Circle

Analyzing access to care and access to research reveals several interrelated equity issues in CAM/TM. Some of them, such as access to care or research funding, are explicitly addressed as equity issues [5, 30]. Other issues were not explicitly identified as equity issues, but can nevertheless be considered as equity issues, e.g. reviewer and publication bias [57, 58]. Procedural issues related to decision-making were described in the PEK context. An attempt to classify the equity issues arising is given in table 1. Some of the equity issues in every dimension are similar to those encountered in other fields of medicine, others are specific to CAM. This is indicated through the references in the right-hand column which refer to CAM-related research and further relevant fields.
Reflecting equity issues arising in the context of CAM, I have identified an anthropological, a policy and a practice dimension. In the present article, the term 'anthropological bias' is used in a different sense than in medical anthropology, where it is described as a feature of anthropological explorations of

Table 1. Equity/Fairness issues in CAM and relevant fields

Dimension of equity	Aspects	Relevant theories
Anthropological dimension	Ideological bias [49] Sponsoring bias [59] Reviewer bias [60] Publication bias [57] Recognition [61] Power [62]	Medical pluralism [21] Cultural imperialism [63]
Policy dimension	Decision-making [64] Priority-setting [65] Power differences [66]	Accountability for reasonableness [64, 66–69]
Practice dimension	Access to care [5] Access to information [13, 15] Medical education [70] Legislation [4, 6, 71] Coverage issues [35, 71, 72]	Concepts of distributive justice [28, 29, 73, 74]

healing [75]. The situation of CAM research within a biomedical context shows an anthropological bias, but quite in the opposite way, as a lack of awareness of medical pluralism and the anthropological and cultural dimension of healing [76, 77]. A common feature of the different kind of bias summarized as anthropological bias in table 1 is the lack of awareness and acknowledgement of the limits of biomedicine and classical biomedical research, as well as of the different ways of thinking about and using evidence across medical traditions and academic disciplines [78].

The second dimension, the 'policy dimension', includes issues related to health policy and decision-making in the context of CAM. These issues are discussed in the first article of this issue and illustrated by the case of PEK. It is noticeable, that the most important fairness issue addressed in PEK, namely the fairness of decision-making, has not yet been addressed in CAM, although the topic is subject to wide debate and an important research topic outside CAM. On the other hand, paradigmatic bias in the PEK context was not perceived as an issue of fairness related to study design but to decision-making.

The third dimension, the 'practice dimension' includes all issues related to the practice of health care. These have mainly been addressed in the section about access to care.

The equity issues are strongly interrelated across these three dimensions. For example, as similarly discussed in the contexts of orphaned fields and primary care, a lack of academic traditions and positions, of research funding, paradigmatic bias and recognition are factors mutually influencing each other. Power relationships within national or international contexts may also have secondary effects on CAM-specific equity issues. For example, current research suggests an important role of pharmaceutical industry as a political player, leading to a situation in which the protection of public health from conventional drugs that are unsafe, unnecessary or ineffective seems to be insufficient [79]. As Abraham points out, 'the pharmaceutical industry has managed not only to gain key positions of influence over drug regulation but also to persuade governments and their regulatory agencies that other interested parties, such as consumer organizations, patients' associations, and the wider medical community, should have few or no rights of access to the regulatory process' [79]. This overall context should be taken into account while discussing safety and effectiveness of CAM. According to Abraham, this situation is particularly striking within the EU. Hence, the difficulties for CAM to be represented by the EU Framework Programmes could also be examined under this aspect [79].

In table 1, an attempt is made to relate the 3 dimensions to different positions and theoretical frameworks [80]. These different approaches to equity and justice reflect, on the one hand, that there is no universal definition of equity and no consensus of its meaning between different academic disciplines dealing with it (philosophy, political theory and economy) [81]. On the other hand, the diversity and multidimensionality of equity issues in CAM needs to be linked to different theoretical approaches. For example, the 'accountability for reasonableness' approach is relevant to investigations and discussions concerning fairness of decision-making. Other justice issues such as the phenomenon of power or the lack of recognition of CAM, i.e. the anthropological bias described above, require other theoretical frameworks that may contribute to the understanding and interpretation of CAM-related equity issues. The specificity of CAM-related questions on equity, justice and fairness are addressed in another article on PEK [82]. That article shows that a health policy decision can be, and in fact was, made against self-declared national and accepted international standards, despite self-professed claims for more fairness and transparency in decision-making, and in the face of contrary empirical PEK study results [1, 22]. Thus, the question arising is: Which theoretical framework contributes to understanding the discrepancy between an increasing body of research (CAM-related issues or issues relevant to CAM), awareness, international standards on the one hand, and the difficulties encountered in doing CAM research, such as the bias described, the lack of recognition and the power differences on the other hand?

Is CAM Facing Cultural Imperialism?

In the last decade awareness of limitations of conventional research methodology and the need to integrate a broad range of evidence increased within conventional medicine. Need for qualified CAM research is also increasing with the growing practice and use of CAM. At the same time, as exemplified in the PEK case, strong resistance in order to prevent such a development exists. Such a resistance may be observed and experienced at all aspects of the equity circle associated with lack of funding, possibilities to carry out research, lack of openness for CAM-related topics in both national and European research funding institutions. An attempt to analyze and understand such a situation shows that concepts of distributive justice, though helpful in order to analyze some of the equity issues arising, do not contribute to a deeper understanding of the situation. As Iris Marion Young points out in her analysis of contemporary American society, many issues of justice do not primarily concern the distribution of material goods but the justice of decision-making power and procedures. In her book 'Justice and the Politics of Difference', she argues that the distributive paradigm neglects the importance of social and institutional contexts and structures, and is not appropriate to represent non-material goods [63]. Young's idea of justice begins with the concept of oppression, a pluralistic concept according to which institutional constraints and social patterns are cutting across individual lives in several ways. The 5 different 'faces of oppression' identified by Young are exploitation, marginalisation, powerlessness, cultural imperialism, and violence. Particularly the concept of cultural imperialism is relevant in CAM contexts, as it involves the 'universalization of a dominant group's experience and culture, and its establishment as the norm'. Due to privileged access in the areas of communication and interpretation, cultural products expressing the values, goals and achievements of the mainstream are widely disseminated, becoming normal and universal. As a consequence, dominant meanings of a society render invisible the particular perspective of one's own group at the same time as they stereotype one's group and mark it out as 'other' [63]. Independently, Fan and Holliday illustrate an example of cultural imperialism in their analysis of medical integration in western China [49]. They demonstrate how the 'all-pervasive' ideology of western science imposes evaluation and reform according to western scientific standards, thereby leading to marginalisation of the traditional medical sector, despite its popularity, and to its fusion with the western medical system [49]. This fusion occurs at different interrelated levels such as education, teaching, the pharmaceutical sector, clinical practice and hospitals, evaluation and regulation. The authors argue for an approach that ensures both traditions to function on a different but equal basis, respecting unique and particular values as well as empirical rules [49].

In western countries, some complementary therapies have their roots in the same culture as conventional medicine. Nonetheless, the patterns described by Young as cultural imperialism, including an interpretation of differences as 'lack and negation' and constructing the different group as 'other' may be observed as well. For example, during the PEK process it could be observed that the label 'alternative medicine' or 'médecine parallèle' was used to construct the 'otherness' of the complementary disciplines assessed, although in daily practice these approaches are in fact a combination and integration of conventional and complementary diagnostic and therapeutic principles. Nevertheless, awareness of this problem seems to increase, as a recent and innovative position of an ethical committee in France reveals, which claims that the term 'alternative' should be avoided, as it implies an attitude of exclusion and lack of tolerance, which may discourage an open dialogue about therapeutic options [83].

Interpreting differences between complementary and conventional approaches as lack and negation are very common in the current controversy about the role of CAM in health care systems: reconsidering them as a consequence of cultural imperialism could foster new and innovative strategies in CAM research. It is commonly assumed that a major obstacle to CAM recognition is the lack of proven effectiveness (according to standards defined in biomedical research), but evidence for this statement itself is not offered. In the ongoing debate about appropriate research methodologies, some authors argue that standards of EBM equally apply to CAM [10]. There is no doubt that such a strategy is necessary, at least in western countries. However, it should include a critical reflection about power differences and patterns that prevent CAM research and recognition. Moreover, claims for applying EBM standards to complementary medicine without reflecting equity issues involved therein may even increase the power differences between CAM and conventional medicine and thus be counterproductive [49]. Furthermore, such claims are frequently made without considering that much of the evidence base for widely accepted conventional therapeutic interventions is at best shaky. This is true in both western countries and countries with strong traditional medical systems such as China [49].

Recent developments of Young's theory of justice reflect discussions that are relevant in the CAM context. For example, McConkey examines problems related to credibility and recognition of marginalized groups. Referring to Wittgenstein's remark that 'knowledge is in the end based on acknowledgement', McConkey highlights the difficulties marginalized groups (e.g. asylum seekers) encounter to be accepted as knowledge claimants and to be credible [61]. She addresses the problem that some knowledge claimants have more credibility than others, and that the process of credibility assessment may benefit groups already privileged or powerful. Similarly, within a medical culture that is dominated by biomedicine, the knowledge claims of those that do not or not entirely belong to the mainstream encounter many difficulties on their way to be acknowledged and recognized as new and valuable knowledge. The difficulty for new CAM-related knowledge to be accepted by the medical establishment is well-known, but the denial of credibility concerning CAM-related knowledge was not yet considered as a concern of justice. An example for such a recognition bias is described by Freeman [84]. At a world conference of family doctors, one of the presented papers examined the holistic attitude of Swedish general practitioners (GPs). In the discussion following the presentation of that paper, it was suggested that one reason why this paper was not eligible for CME credit was that the programme committee presumed the paper to be about alternative medicine (associated with holism), thus not scientific and thus unworthy of CME credit. It is noteworthy that this situation was not described in a specialized CAM journal or article.

Discussing the concept of cultural imperialism with respect to CAM, it is important to remember that anthropological as well as recognition bias seem to be characteristic for the situation of CAM in western countries. In contrast, the official recognition of traditional medicine is widespread among developing countries. Here it is sometimes officially supported as it is part of the cultural heritage and considered useful for low-income countries where access to modern pharmaceuticals is lacking [85–87].

Concluding Remarks

Although a global approach to equity issues considered in the context of medical pluralism would require further clarification and exploration, several equity issues arising with the increasing use of TM/CAM were identified. Inequities related to access to care can be observed in industrialized countries. Further discrimination results from the strong influence of industry on trials, guidelines and education. Considering the equity issues addressed in this paper from a global perspective, we may notice both common and different trends in industrialized and developing countries. Whereas the equity issues related to research (due to the dominant paradigm and lack of funding) are similar in industrialized and developing countries, we can observe opposite trends in these two types of countries with respect to access to care, health policy and public recognition. However, public recognition of TM/CAM, or the lack of recognition, seems to be ideology driven in industrialized as well as in developing countries. In industrialized countries, the lack of public recognition is associated with the dominance of biomedicine and the respective political and economical powers; in developing countries TM is recognized as part of their cultural heritage. Also, the cost argument seems to be strongly associated with value judgements: in industrialized countries the cost argument is brought to argue against CAM, whereas in developing countries the opposite happens, TM is considered cheaper as western medicine, which is often not accessible to the majority of the population. Therefore, medical pluralism may offer some broader perspectives and encourage policy makers to learn from other countries with the aim to offer patients the 'best of both worlds' and to reduce inequities.

A classification was proposed consisting of three main dimensions (anthropological, policy and practice) which were linked to different theoretical frameworks. While two of these theoretical approaches (the distributive paradigm and the 'accountability for reasonableness' framework) were discussed in a precedent article, the present article demonstrates the relevance of Youngs' understanding of justice and concept of cultural imperialism for the phenomenon of power observed in the context of CAM.

The global perspective chosen here in order to discuss equity issues of CAM/TM is associated with several major problems that lead to certain weaknesses of this article. (1) It is difficult to define CAM/TM. Hence, I have used the broad definition according to the WHO. However, access to care and coverage issues have to be discussed on the basis of specific CAM definitions relevant in the context of national health care systems. (2) There is no universal theory of equity and justice. Different paradigms and a lack of agreement, even within the distributive paradigm, about what should be equal make universal arguments difficult [81]. (3) Linking theoretical concepts of equity with the practice and policy dimension is debatable [81]. Yet, the diversity of theoretical approaches to equity also offers concepts that are appropriate to the multidimensionality of CAM-related equity issues. As this article may show, the contribution of political science as a discipline is relevant in contexts of CAM. It particularly contributes to interpreting anthropological and ideological factors associated with CAM/TM in both industrialized and developing countries, albeit in some different ways.

The given interrelatedness of equity issues implies the acknowledgment that changes in one of the dimensions have implications on the others, from a global as well as from a long-term perspective. The complexity of the 'equity circle' requires further research which should combine empirical and theoretical approaches including distributive issues, fairness in processes and procedures, as well as approaches that contribute to understanding anthropological and societal dimensions of equity and justice in different contexts of CAM. CAM requires understanding and claims for fairness in a distributive sense (non-discrimination of health care delivery, funding, academic positions) and claims for a positive valorisation of identity and diversity.

The concept of medical pluralism is a key concept that allows for a discussion of CAM-related issues from a broader and global perspective. Medical pluralism may address the diversity of healing cultures that exist alongside biomedicine all over the world, and is the research field of medical anthropology. While cultural imperialism has been the subject of a wide critical reflection in the fields of political and social sciences, this debate seems not to have been taken into account within mainstream medicine and by policy makers, nor has a reflection taken place comparable to other fields.

Two out of four principles of biomedical ethics have been considered in this article: respect for autonomy (as closely related to the recognition of medical pluralism) and justice. Further research should strive to better integrate and examine these two principles in the ongoing debates on CAM, which are often unduly limited to a discussion about effectiveness, which is only one aspect of beneficence.

Acknowledgements

This study was supported by the Stiftung Merkur-Rafael, the Fondation Homéopathique Pierre Schmidt and the University of Bern. I thank Heather Murray, Klaus von Ammon, Bryn Williams- Jones and Johan Hulson for their comments on an earlier draft of this paper. I thank Harald Walach for the review of this manuscript.

References

1 WHO (ed): Fact Sheet No 134, 2003. Geneva, World Health Organization, 2003.
2 WHO (ed): WHO Global Atlas of Traditional, Complementary and Alternative medicine. Kobe, WHO Centre of Health Development, 2005.
3 Adams KE, Cohen MH, Eisenberg D, Jonsen AR: Ethical considerations of complementary and alternative medical therapies in conventional medical settings. Ann Intern Med 2002;137:660–664.
4 Cohen MH: Legal and ethical issues in complementary medicine: a United States perspective. Med J Aust 2004;181:168–169.
5 Ernst E, Cohen MH, Stone J: Ethical problems arising in evidence based complementary and alternative medicine. J Med Ethics 2004;30:156–159.
6 Cohen MH: Legal and ethical issues relating to use of complementary therapies in pediatric hematology/oncology. J Pediatr Hematol Oncol 2006;28:190–193.
7 Cohen MH, Eisenberg DM: Potential physician malpractice liability associated with complementary and integrative medical therapies. Ann Intern Med 2002;136:596–603.
8 Kerridge IH, McPhee JR: Ethical and legal issues at the interface of complementary and conventional medicine. Med J Aust 2004;181:164–166.
9 Zuck R: [Evaluation and pluralism from the viewpoint of constitutional law]. Z Arztl Fortbild Qualitatssich 2005;99:263–267.
10 Miller FG, Emanuel EJ, Rosenstein DL, Straus SE: Ethical issues concerning research in complementary and alternative medicine. Jama 2004;291:599–604.
11 Kaptchuk TJ, Lembo A: Ethical issues in research in complementary and alternative medicine. Jama 2004;291:2193; author reply 2193–2194.
12 Sugarman J: Informed consent, shared decision-making, and complementary and alternative medicine. J Law Med Ethics 2003;31:247–250.
13 Sugarman J, Burk L: Physicians' ethical obligations regarding alternative medicine. Jama 1998;280:1623–1625.
14 Caspi O, Holexa J: Lack of standards in informed consent in complementary and alternative medicine. Complement Ther Med 2005;13:123–130.
15 Brophy E: Does a doctor have a duty to provide information and advice about complementary and alternative medicine? J Law Med 2003;10:271–284.
16 Ernst E, Cohen MH: Informed consent in complementary and alternative medicine. Arch Intern Med 2001;161:2288–2292.
17 Höffe O: Gerechtigkeit. Eine philosophische Einführung. München, Beck, 2004.
18 Beauchamp TL, Childress JF: Principles of Biomedical Ethics, ed 5. Oxford, Oxford University Press, 2001.
19 Kiene H, Ollenschlager G, Willich SN: [Pluralism in medicine – pluralism or therapeutic evaluation?]. Z Arztl Fortbild Qualitatssich 2005;99:261–262.
20 Bensing J: Bridging the gap. The separate worlds of evidence-based medicine and patient-centered medicine. Patient Educ Couns 2000;39:17–25.
21 Institute of Medicine (ed): Complementary and Alternative Medicine in the United States. IOM, 2005.
22 WHO (ed): WHO traditional medicine strategy 2002–2005. Geneva, World Health Organization, 2002.
23 WHO (ed): Traditional Medicine Fact Sheet No 134, 2003. Geneva, World Health Organization, 2003.
24 Berman BM: Integrative approaches to pain management: how to get the best of both worlds. BMJ 2003;326:1320a–1321.
25 Charles PW: The best of both worlds. BMJ 2001; 322:181.
26 Barrett B: Alternative, complementary, and conventional medicine: is integration upon us? J Altern Complement Med 2003;9:417–427.
27 Kaptchuk TJ, Miller FG: Viewpoint: what is the best and most ethical model for the relationship between mainstream and alternative medicine: opposition, integration, or pluralism? Acad Med 2005; 80:286–290.
28 Sen A: Why health equity? Health Econ 2002;11:659–666.
29 Alkire S, Chen L: Global health and moral values. Lancet 2004;364:1069–1074.
30 Stone J, Matthews J: Complementary medicine and the law. Oxford, Oxford University Press, 1996.
31 Fisher P, van Haselen R, Hardy K, Berkovitz S, McCarney R: Effectiveness gaps: a new concept for evaluating health service and research needs applied to complementary and alternative medicine. J Altern Complement Med 2004;10:627–632.
32 Braveman P, Gruskin S: Defining equity in health. J Epidemiol Community Health 2003;57:254–258.
33 Marian F, Widmer M, Herren S, Donges A, Busato A: Physicians' philosophy of care: a comparison of complementary and conventional medicine. Forsch Komplementarmed 2006;13:70–77.
34 Gottlieb S: One in three doctors don't tell patients about services they can't have. BMJ 2003;327:123-a.
35 Wynia MK, VanGeest JB, Cummins DS, Wilson IB: Do physicians not offer useful services because of coverage restrictions? Health Aff (Millwood) 2003; 22:190–197.
36 Slowther A, Ford S, Schofield T: Ethics of evidence based medicine in the primary care setting. J Med Ethics 2004;30:151–155.
37 ten Have H: Ethical perspectives on health technology assessment. Int J Technol Assess Health Care 2004;20:71–76.
38 Heusser P: [Criteria for assessing benefit with complementary medical methods]. Forsch Komplementarmed Klass Naturheilkd 2001;8:14–23.
39 Kienle GS: [Is there a rationale for pluralistic evaluation models? Limitations of randomized clinical trials]. Z Arztl Fortbild Qualitatssich 2005;99:289–294.
40 Starfield B: New paradigms for quality in primary care. Br J Gen Pract 2001;51:303–309.
41 Walach H, Falkenberg T, Fonnebo V, Lewith G, Jonas WB: Circular instead of hierarchical: methodological principles for the evaluation of complex interventions. BMC Med Res Methodol 2006;6:29.
42 Crivelli L: Slimming diet for the FHIA benefit basket; in Monitor HP (ed): Lugano, Università della Svizzera Italiana, 2005.
43 Walach H: The Swiss Program for the Evaluation of Complementary Medicine (PEK). J Altern Complement Med 2006;12:231–232.
44 Walach H, Linde K, Eichenberger R, Stalder H, Kristensen FB, Kleijnen J: Summary consensus statement of the PEK Review Board regarding the PEK process and the PEK products. J Altern Complement Med 2006;12:347–348.
45 Abramson J, Starfield B: The effect of conflict of interest on biomedical research and clinical practice guidelines: Can we trust the evidence in evidence-based medicine? J Am Board Fam Pract 2005;18:414–418.
46 Rogers WA: Evidence based medicine and justice: a framework for looking at the impact of EBM upon vulnerable or disadvantaged groups. J Med Ethics 2004;30:141–145.
47 Vos R, Willems D, Houtepen R: Coordinating the norms and values of medical research, medical practice and patient worlds – the ethics of evidence based medicine in orphaned fields of medicine. J Med Ethics 2004;30:166–170.
48 Critchley JA, Zhang Y, Suthisisang CC, Chan TY, Tomlinson B: Alternative therapies and medical science: designing clinical trials of alternative/complementary medicines – is evidence-based traditional Chinese medicine attainable? J Clin Pharmacol 2000;40:462–467.
49 Fan R, Holliday I: Which medicine? Whose standard? Critical reflections on medical integration in China. J Med Ethics 2007;33:454–461.
50 Gotzsche PC: Research integrity and pharmaceutical industry sponsorship. Trial registration, transparency and less reliance on industry trials are essential. Med J Aust 2005;182:549–550.
51 Lewith GT, Bensoussan A: Complementary and alternative medicine – with a difference. Med J Aust 2004;180:585–586.

52 Lewith GT: Complementary and alternative medicine: an educational, attitudinal and research challenge. Med J Aust 2000;172:102–103.
53 Ernst E: Only 0.08% of funding for research in NHS goes to complementary medicine. BMJ 1996; 313:882-b.
54 Witt C, Keil T, Selim D, Roll S, Vance W, Wegscheider K, Willich SN: Outcome and costs of homoeopathic and conventional treatment strategies: a comparative cohort study in patients with chronic disorders. Complement Ther Med 2005;13:79–86.
55 Hamre HJ, Becker-Witt C, Glockmann A, Ziegler R, Willich SN, Kiene H: Anthroposophic therapies in chronic disease: the Anthroposophic Medicine Outcomes Study (AMOS). Eur J Med Res 2004;9: 351–360.
56 Menniti-Ippolito F, Gargiulo L, Bologna E, Forcella E, Raschetti R: Use of unconventional medicine in Italy: a nation-wide survey. Eur J Clin Pharmacol 2002;58:61–64.
57 Vannacci A, Ravaldi C, Cosci F: Publication bias in complementary and conventional medicine. Eur J Clin Pharmacol 2005;61:161–162; author reply 163.
58 Ernst E, Resch KL: Reviewer bias against the unconventional? A randomized double-blind study of peer review. Complement Ther Med 1999;7:19–23.
59 Abraham J: Bias in science and medical knowledge: the Opren controversy. Sociology 1994;28: 717–736.
60 Resch KI, Ernst E, Garrow J: A randomized controlled study of reviewer bias against an unconventional therapy. J R Soc Med 2000;93:164–167.
61 McConkey J: Knowledge and Acknowledgement: 'Epistemic injustice' as a problem of recognition. Politics 2004;24:198–205.
62 Heusser P: Medizin und Macht am Beispiel des Programms Evaluation Komplementärmedizin PEK; in Ausfeld-Hafter B (ed): Medizin und Macht. Die Arzt-Patienten-Beziehung im Wandel: Mehr Entscheidungsfreiheit? Bern, Peter Lang, 2007.
63 Young IM: Justice and the Politics of Difference. Princeton, NJ, Princeton University Press, 1990.
64 Daniels N, Sabin J: The ethics of accountability in managed care reform. Health Aff (Millwood) 1998; 17:50–64.
65 Peacock S, Ruta D, Mitton C, Donaldson C, Bate A, Murtagh M: Using economics to set pragmatic and ethical priorities. BMJ 2006;332:482–485.
66 Gibson JL, Martin DK, Singer PA: Priority setting in hospitals: fairness, inclusiveness, and the problem of institutional power differences. Soc Sci Med 2005;61:2355–2362.
67 Gibson JL, Martin DK, Singer PA: Setting priorities in health care organizations: criteria, processes, and parameters of success. BMC Health Serv Res 2004;4:25.
68 Gibson JL, Martin DK, Singer PA: Priority setting for new technologies in medicine: a transdisciplinary study. BMC Health Serv Res 2002;2:14.
69 Martin DK, Giacomini M, Singer PA: Fairness, accountability for reasonableness, and the views of priority setting decision-makers. Health Policy 2002;61:279–290.
70 Park CM: Diversity, the individual, and proof of efficacy: complementary and alternative medicine in medical education. Am J Public Health 2002;92: 1568–1572.
71 Ersdal G: How are patients safeguarded when using complementary and alternative medicine (CAM)? Jurisdiction, supervision and reimbursement status in the EEA area (EU and EFTA) and Switzerland; in CAM-Cancer project funded by the EU Commission within the FP 5 Quality of life. 2005.
72 Crivelli L: Slimming diet for the FHIA benefit basket; in Health Policy Monitor. Lugano, Universita della Svizzera Italiana, 2005.
73 Aristoteles: Nikomachische Ethik. Stuttgart, Reclam, 1969.
74 Horn C, Scarano N (eds): Philosophie der Gerechtigkeit. Texte von der Antike bis zur Gegenwart. Frankfurt/M., Suhrkamp, 2002.
75 Bolton J: Medical practice and anthropological bias. Soc Sci Med 1995;40:1655–1661.
76 Good BJ: Medicina, racionalidad y experiencia. Una perspectiva antropológica. Barcelona, Bellaterra, 2003.
77 Kirmayer LJ: The cultural diversity of healing: meaning, metaphor and mechanism. Br Med Bull 2004;69:33–48.
78 De Vries R: (Bio)Ethics and evidence: from collaboration to co-operation; in Gastmans C, Dierickx K, Nys H, Schotmans P (eds): New Pathways for European Bioethics. Antwerpen, Intersentia, 2007.
79 Abraham J: The pharmaceutical industry as a political player. Lancet 2002;360:1498–1502.
80 Alkire S, Chen L: Global health and moral values. Lancet 2004;364:1069–1074.
81 Culyer AJ: Equity – some theory and its policy implications. J Med Ethics 2001;27:275–283.
82 Marian F: Complementary medicine: equity issues in evaluation and policy-making. Forsch Komplementarmed 2007;6(suppl 2):2–9.
83 Commission d'éthique (ed): A médecines multiples, devoir médical unique; in Bulletin de l'Ordre. Ordre départemental des médecins de Côte d'Or. Dijon, 2007.
84 Freeman J: Towards a definition of holism. Br J Gen Pract 2005;55:154–155.
85 Sydara K, Gneunphonsavath S, Wahlstrom R, Freudenthal S, Houamboun K, Tomson G, Falkenberg T: Use of traditional medicine in Lao PDR. Complement Ther Med 2005;13:199–205.
86 Bodeker G: Lessons on integration from the developing world's experience. BMJ 2001;322:164–167.
87 Tsey K: Traditional medicine in contemporary Ghana: a public policy analysis. Soc Sci Med 1997; 45:1065–1074.

Forschende Komplementärmedizin
Wissenschaft • Praxis • Perspektiven

Original Article · Originalarbeit

Forsch Komplementärmed 2007;14(suppl 2):19–27
DOI: 10.1159/000112455

Exploring Different Dimensions of Holism: Considerations in the Context of an Evaluation of Complementary Medicine in Primary Care

Florica Marian

Institute for Complementary Medicine KIKOM, University of Bern, Switzerland

Key Words
Holism · Integrative medicine · Complementary medicine · Health technology assessment · Evaluation · Primary care

Summary
Holism is often associated with both complementary medicine and primary care. In the context of the Swiss Programme for the Evaluation of Complementary Medicine (PEK), the concept of holism emerged from data on physician's philosophy of care and motivation for patients' choice of physician. Yet, as PEK primarily aimed to quantify differences between conventional and complementary medicine, qualitative aspects of the study were neglected and data not fully explored. The main objective of this article is to explore the concept, variations and dimensions of holism by exploring and reflecting on PEK results implicitly and explicitly related to holism.

Schlüsselwörter
Holismus · Ganzheitlichkeit · Integrative Medizin · Komplementärmedizin · Health Technology Assessment · Evaluation · Grundversorgung

Zusammenfassung
Ganzheitlichkeit wird oft mit Komplementärmedizin und Grundversorgung in Verbindung gebracht. Im Kontext des Schweizerischen Programms Evaluation Komplementärmedizin (PEK) wurde Ganzheitlichkeit als wesentliche Komponente sowohl der ärztlichen Versorgungsphilosophie als auch der Patientenmotivation in der Komplementärmedizin erfasst. Da die PEK-Studien jedoch vor allem das Ziel hatten, Unterschiede zwischen konventioneller Medizin und Komplementärmedizin zu quantifizieren, wurden qualitative Aspekte der Studien vernachlässigt und die Daten in dieser Hinsicht nicht ausgewertet. In diesem Artikel sollen das Konzept Ganzheitlichkeit sowie Variationen und Dimensionen von Ganzheitlichkeit beleuchtet werden. Dazu werden Ergebnisse der PEK-Studien exploriert und reflektiert, die implizit oder explizit mit Ganzheitlichkeit zusammenhängen.

Introduction

Holism is a concept which is often associated with complementary and alternative medicine (CAM) and also, increasingly, with primary care. In the context of a health technology assessments (HTA) of complementary medicine, the Swiss Programme for the Evaluation of Complementary Medicine (PEK), the concept of holism emerged from data on physician's philosophy of care and motivation for patients' choice of physicians [1, 2]. Yet, as the PEK study primarily aimed to quantify differences between conventional and complementary medicine, qualitative aspects of the study were neglected and data not fully explored. The main objective of this article is to explore the concept, variations and dimensions of holism by examining qualitative PEK data. Further objectives are to discuss the implications of those results for health policy issues related to complementary medicine.

The term 'holism' is very often used but rarely defined. This may be due to the complexity of the concept and its roots. First, it is connected with the Greek term 'holos' (whole), and

KARGER

Fax +49 761 4 52 07 14
E-mail Information@Karger.de
www.karger.com

Accessible online at:
www.karger.com/fok

Dr. rer. med. Florica Marian, lic. phil.
Kollegiale Instanz für Komplementärmedizin KIKOM
Universität Bern, Inselspital Imhoof Pavillon
CH-3010 Bern, Switzerland
Tel. +41 31 6328606, Fax 6324262
E-mail florence.marian@kikom.unibe.ch

one of the very first definitions was given within the context of geography by Jan Christian Smuts [1926], who followed Aristotle: 'The whole is not a mechanical system. It consists indeed of parts, but it is more than the sum of its parts, which a purely mechanical system necessarily is. A whole, which is more than the sum of its parts, has something internal, some inwardness of structure and function, some specific inner relations, some internality of character or nature which constitutes that more'. A similar definition was introduced in 1980 in the PubMed database: 'Health as viewed from the perspective that humans and other organisms function as complete, integrated units rather than as aggregates of separate parts' [3]. Other approaches consider holism from a much broader perspective in connection with the concepts of health and healing. Walach [4] considers the Indo-German common root 'hal' for a family of concepts including 'heil' and 'heilig' (German), 'whole', 'holy', 'hallow', and possibly also the Greek 'hagios' (holy) and 'hygieia' (health). Boyd [5] addresses the interconnectedness of wholeness and healing from a religious perspective, according to which healing is not only understood 'as the natural process of tissue regeneration sometimes assisted by medical means, but also as whatever process results in the experience of greater wholeness of the human spirit. Healing in the latter sense need not be religious in form (nature, music or friendship as well as religious rites may be agents of healing), nor accompanied by "cures" or "miracles". These or other signs of hope, when attested, may be seen as traces of a transcendent or encompassing wholeness, in which human wholeness is grounded. But wholeness is always imperfectly realised in the fragmentariness of human experience: and while for religion the encompassing is not reducible to a psychological projection, it is discovered most commonly in the mode of expectancy, both in the midst of life and in the face of death.' Though often associated with complementary medicine, holism is increasingly considered as relevant in conventional medicine and particularly in primary care [6]. Nonetheless, it is important to remember that holism is neither specific to complementary medicine nor a modern phenomenon but rather an essential dimension in Plato's philosophy and Hippocratic medicine [7, 8]. A definition of Plato's understanding of holism is given in 'Charmides': 'This Thracian told me that in these notions of theirs, which I was just now mentioning, the Greek physicians are quite right as far as they go, but Zalmoxis, he added, our king, who is also a god, says further "that as you ought not to attempt to cure the eyes without the head, or the head without the body, so neither ought you to attempt to cure the body without the soul." And this, he said, "is the cause why the cure of many diseases is unknown to the physicians of Hellas, because they disregard the whole (to holon), which ought to be studied also, for the part (to meros) can never be well unless the whole is well. For all good and evil, whether in the body or in the whole man, originates", as he declared, "in the soul, and overflows from thence, as if from the head into the eyes. And therefore if the head and body are to be well, you must begin by curing the soul – that is the first and essential thing"' [9, pp 156d6–157a3].

Furthermore, some current approaches to medical ethics that emphasize the contribution of philosophy (e.g. Paul Ricoeur and Emmanuel Levinas) to an ethics of care can be considered holistic [10]. Despite a broad consensus on the importance of holism in CAM, little attention has been given to explore and describe this concept. In fact, as current developments show, holism seems to be increasingly investigated in primary conventional care [3, 11, 12]. This leads to questions about differences between the understanding of holism in conventional and complementary medicine, and about the integration of both approaches by overcoming thinking in dichotomies [4]. On this background, the present article aims to promote debate and reflection about holism.

The article is structured as follows: The first section gives a brief introduction into current discussions about holism, focusing on complementary medicine and primary care. The second part, explores the dimensions of holism on the basis of the PEK studies. The third part discusses possible consequences for ethical, policy and research issues as well as possible differences between the conception of holism in conventional and complementary medicine.

Holism: Key Issues in Current Discussions

The significance of holism in health care is discussed in several distinct but related fields: complementary medicine, primary care, nursing and philosophy of medicine. According to the aims of this article, I will outline some aspects of these discussions in complementary medicine and primary care.

Complementary Medicine

The significance of holistic values is well documented in the CAM literature [2, 13–17]. Holistic values have been described as a main predictor of CAM use [18]. Holistic health has been identified as one of three distinct dimensions associated with CAM use and has been integrated in the holistic CAM questionnaire [19]. Holism is considered a core component of CAM (like the notions of self-healing and a systems approach to health) [17]. In general, the term holism is very often used in CAM and comprises a broad variety of meanings and significations. Barrett et al. [14] for example, subsume the following concepts under holism: acceptance, community, continuity, empathy, energetics, feedback, healing, health maintenance, integration, knowing your body, listening to one's self, mind-body unity, open-mindedness, practice style, prevention, psychological, spirituality, unbroken, uniqueness. Besides the general aspect of treating the whole person (body, mind and spirit) within their environment, Long, too, distinguishes several aspects and perspectives [17]: interconnectedness between patient, practitioner and environment, treatment at all levels or the conviction that treatment at one level

Table 1. Qualitative PEK data used and actual status of analysis / publication

Data from PEK questionnaires	Status
Physicians	
Questionnaire about structural characteristics of practises	
1. What are the convictions and values that provide the basis of your medical activities or the application of particular diagnostic or therapeutic procedures?	
2. Please describe which priorities you set in your medical activity	
3. If you are using complementary medicine, what was the motivation to start working with it?	
4. you are using both conventional and complementary medicine, what are your criteria of choice?	1.–5. Partly analyzed and published [2]
5. Where do you see the limitations of the methods applied?	
6. Did you observe some changes since you are practising complementary medicine?	6. Not analyzed; not published
Patients	
Questionnaire at consultation	
7. For which reasons have you chosen this physician?	7. Analyzed; report unpublished [25]

has consequences at all levels, a systemic understanding of illness as imbalance and a corresponding and individualized approach to treatment [17]. Further approaches focus on the holistic character of health [4, 16, 20] and consider health and illness as related to 'holistic togetherness' at organic, social and natural (within the whole of nature) levels [20]. Holism also plays a role in discussions about relevant outcome measures in CAM: acknowledging the whole systems approach of care which characterizes many CAM interventions requires holistic outcomes that encompass physical, psychological, social and spiritual dimensions [21].

Primary Care

The incorporation of holistic values into conventional medicine and especially into primary care is considered as particular step in the development of medicine [14, 22]. The emergence of holistic thinking is associated with criticism on the reductionism of modern medicine with its focus on technology and laboratory research and its lack of concern for the whole patient [22], and also with a paradigmatic change from a biomedical to a patient-centred approach in medicine [6, 22]. According to Goldstein et al. [23], 'holistic health' and 'holistic medicine' were frequently used to characterize primary care in the United States, although the concept had not been clearly defined. In the meantime, current developments show that holism is increasingly defined and empirically investigated in primary care. For example, 'holistic modelling' is one of the 6 core competencies of the general practitioner (GP) and defined as 'the ability to use a biopsychosocial model taking into account cultural and existential dimensions' as well as the ability to deal with health problems in their physical, psychological, social, cultural and existential dimensions' (European Academy of Teachers in General Practice Euract, 2002) [3]. Such an approach to health and disease seems to be widely shared among GPs: 'We are not doctors for particular diseases, or particular organs, or particular stages in the life cycle – we are doctors for people' [11]. Furthermore, 'everything affects health, and as physicians dedicated to maintaining and improving health we must understand and honour the whole, in each of its parts and with the synergies that are created as they act together' [11]. In Sweden, too, holism is considered a core concept in primary care (with quality, accessibility, continuity and collaboration) [3]. Accordingly, all aspects of people's needs, be they psychological, physical or social, should be considered and seen as a whole [3]. A similar definition can be found in the WHO Charta for General Practice according to which holistic signifies the physical, psychological, and social perspective of individuals, families and communities [3].

In a recent qualitative study on the meaning of personal care in general practice, three main features of personal care were identified: human communication, individualized or tailored care, and 'whole person' or holistic care [12]. A holistic attitude is expected by patients in general practice [24].

In the context of the increasing recognition of holism as a core dimension of primary care, questions arise about differences and similarities between holistic aspects of complementary medicine and primary care. Some authors assume that such differences exist, and propose to use the term 'wholistic' in primary care and the term 'holistic' in CAM [3]. While this approach (based on a qualitative study conducted in Swedish primary care [3]) assumes that primary care and CAM do not have much in common, experiences and results in the context of the PEK studies allow to explore holism within a health system that integrates some complementary therapies into primary care.

Finally, holism is considered as a core dimension in nursing. It is defined in the PubMed database as 'a philosophy of nursing practice that takes into account total patient care, considering

Table 2. Patients' reasons for the choice of their general practitioner

Patient reasons (AM GP) n = 688 patients (≥16 years)	Patient reasons (conventional GP) n = 3,078 patients (≥16 years)
Specific methods wanted (19.8%)	Family doctor (33.8%)
Holistic treatment (17.1%)	Competence/truthfulness of GP (24.5%)
Competence/truthfulness of GP (16.9%)	Illness (9.7%)
Recommendation (8.2%)	Geographic proximity (7.9%)
Family doctor (7.8%)	Recommendation (6.5%)
Personal conviction (7.2%)	Control and check-up (3.7%)
Mild treatment (4.9%)	Others (13.9%)
Illness (3.9%)	
Dissatisfaction with conventional medicine (3.0%)	
Others (12%)	

AM = Anthroposophic medicine.
GP = General practitioner.

the physical, emotional, social, economic, and spiritual needs of patients, their response to their illnesses, and the effect of illness on patients' abilities to meet self-care needs' [3].

Dimensions of Holism in the PEK Studies

Questions about a possible contribution of the PEK studies to an exploration of the concept of holism were raised at different instances: (1) during the PEK study about physicians' philosophy of care [2], (2) when considering PEK data about the changes physicians had observed as a consequence of the practice of complementary medicine, and (3) when considering PEK data on the motivation of patients' choice of physicians [25]. In the PEK studies themselves no question directly focussed on holism. Nevertheless, the answers physicians and patients gave to several questions show that holism is a core component of complementary medicine both in physicians and in patients (table 1).
Concerning physicians, only the results related to questions 1–5 have been published to date [2]; data concerning question 6 have not yet been analyzed. According to the political aim of the PEK studies, the study on physicians' philosophy of care focussed on quantifiable differences between complementary and conventional medicine, and therefore neglected the qualitative character of the study [2]. Patient-related data is given in a PEK report [25]. The analysis and publication of the huge amount of data collected during PEK was associated with major difficulties that are described elsewhere [26–29]. As a consequence of the attitude of the responsible authorities since 2004, part of the data has not been analyzed, interpreted, reflected and/or published until now. This is important to know in order to understand the difference between the sources used for the present article and their differing status with respect to the disciplines concerned and with respect to previous analyses and publications (table 1). These sources include: (1) Data collected in the questionnaire on structural characteristics of practices (including philosophy of care), which have been partly analyzed and published (i.e. anthroposophic medicine (AM), homeopathy, neural therapy and traditional Chinese medicine) [2], (2) patient data collected at consultation and analyzed in an unpublished report (AM) [25].

Holistic Treatment as Dimension of Patient Motivation in CAM

PEK data suggest that the reasons to see a GP are different in complementary and conventional medicine. Table 2 presents the differences described in a PEK report on AM [25].
Summarizing the different aspects mentioned by the patients into the dimensions physician-related / procedures-related / pragmatic reasons, we can observe that in conventional medicine, pragmatic reasons are mentioned most frequently (61.9%), followed by physician-related (36.7%) and procedures-related reasons (2.4%). In AM, however, reasons related to methods/procedures are mentioned most frequently (49.1%), followed by physician-related (32.0%) and pragmatic reasons (18.9%). The importance of holistic treatment approaches for patients who seek complementary medicine is well known and has been repeatedly described in the CAM literature [13, 18]. The importance of holism is also increasingly documented in conventional care, but this could possibly not be measured in our questionnaire that asked patients the reasons for seeking their GP.

Dimensions of Holism Arising in Physicians' Philosophy of Care

While the PEK patient data reveal the importance of holism to their motivation for the choice of their GP, the PEK physician answers (table 1) allow deeper insights into the phenomenon of holism itself at two levels. First, holism as an overall

Table 3. A 4-dimensional approach to holism

Dimension of holism	Aspects
Wholeness of patient	Awareness of physical, emotional, social and spiritual needs of patients Awareness of patient responsibility, freedom, autonomy Awareness of sense and meaning of health and illness
Wholeness of physician	Find sense and meaning in professional activity Satisfaction with profession associated with: joy, quality of life, better health (no burnout), less side effects, better relationship to environment Therapeutic freedom
Integration of therapeutic approaches	Synthesis of complementary and conventional approaches Awareness of limits of conventional, complementary approaches and for individual limits of patient and physician Individual combination of self-regulatory, preventive, resource-oriented and curative approaches
Relational dimension	Therapeutic attitude respectful towards environment Quality of perception and relations to human, social, natural, spiritual environments Importance of communication

characteristic of physicians' philosophy of care in complementary medicine was a category that emerged from the data [2]. The category 'holism' was applied to all answers that referred to an interrelatedness of body, mind and spirit or to the multidimensionality of the patient and therapeutic situation (opposed to a positivistic worldview). In the present article, I will explore different dimensions of holism on the basis of physicians' philosophy of care, therefore, the methodology is different from that in the first study [2]. In that previous study, key issues were identified, i.e. concepts and themes by means of which the data could be examined and referenced. Categories were constructed and refined at first, in order to reflect as many nuances of the data as possible; only then, these categories were reduced by combination and by forming main and subcategories [2]. Holism was a main category to characterize the worldview, as opposed to a positivistic outlook. In the present article, however, I have started from the concept of holism, searching for variations of this phenomenon both in PEK data and the literature. The choice for this strategy, which is characteristic for phenomenological approaches [30], was influenced by two factors: (1) Due to the political aim of the PEK study (determine and quantify differences between conventional and complementary medicine), the qualitative aspect (variety of individual answers) was neglected in the first data analysis and in the interpretation of physicians' philosophy of care [2]. (2) Due to methodological weaknesses of the PEK studies (lack of validation and pre-testing of questionnaires), some questions were answered differently. For example, the question about priorities was either understood as a question about the medical specialty practised, or as a question about the focus within the consultation, or as a question about values. This lack of focus and specificity in the questions was associated with a broad variety in physicians' answers. A re-examination of physician data (table 1) with respect to holism revealed four main dimensions: wholeness of patient, wholeness of physician, relational dimension and therapeutic approaches (table 3).

Wholeness of Patient

Different perspectives on wholeness of patients are reflected in the answers of physicians, e.g. theoretical frameworks such as the biopsychosocial model, Christian values, Chinese philosophy or anthroposophy. (A somehow different level, yet still connected with the wholeness of patients, is the gender dimension, CAM being considered as better appropriate to the needs of women.)

Examples of physicians' answers:

(1) 'The human being is a whole. When she seeks help, she needs understanding for her personality with all her aspects, for her illness, symptoms as well as for her emotional and social needs. Diagnostics and therapy must take these aspects into account.'

(2) 'The human being is on a path determined by his karma, reincarnation, genealogy, education and possibility to freedom. In these woven elements, illness has a deeper meaning with respect to the individual person and a meaning for him and his environment ...'

(3) 'My patients feel more responsible for themselves, since we have talked about such connections between life, nutrition and prevention.'

Wholeness of Physician

Physicians' free-text answers to the question about changes since they started practising complementary medicine express better overall satisfaction with their profession and better quality of life. Better satisfaction was not related to holism by the physicians themselves, but the terms in which they described it show that the practice of CAM helps physicians be and consider themselves as a whole. This dimension was mainly related to the motivation for the practice of CAM and to changes through the practice of CAM (table 1, questions 3 and 6).

Examples of physicians' answers:

(1) 'Dissatisfaction with materialistic models of sciences and medicine, search for deeper understanding and meaning in everything that occurs (e.g. Viktor Frankl). Possibility to find a therapeutic attitude that is highly respectful towards human beings and environment.'
(2) 'My relationship to people has tremendously increased, my attention has improved, my 'antennas' for human beings, animals and nature have become more sensitive, and I have found more intensity and joy in life. My quality of life has become more meaningful and harmonized.'
(3) 'Enjoying being a general practitioner – no burnout – less side-effects in therapy – great motivation of patients.'
(4) 'I experience more meaning and sense in my professional activity: satisfaction is more than money and reputation.'

Wholeness as Integration of Therapeutic Approaches

An integrative approach that combines conventional and complementary medicine is clearly reflected in the physicians' answers (table 1) and can be considered as holistic. Such an integrative approach is multidimensional, i.e. it encompasses a deeper understanding of illness and its meanings, looks not only at symptoms but also at causes and meanings and is aware of limits (both therapeutic and personal limits) and the individual combination of self-regulatory, preventive, resource-oriented and curative approaches.

Examples:

(1) 'Every patient is unique regarding his biography. My aim is to care for every patient in her totality. Illnesses are syndromes whose origin has to be found individually for every single patient. Headaches, for example, may have 10 different causes in 10 different patients.
(2) 'I consider myself as a conventional physician that uses softer methods, helping patients develop their self-healing energies (with classical homeopathy, psychotherapy and Rolfing). It is essential to find out when patients have enough energy, and to this end complementary medicine is appropriate, and when they need external energy. Both complementary and conventional medicine should be self-critical and not dogmatic, because they complement each other within an 'integrative medicine'. I understand healing as daily actualization of health and consider myself as a disciple of salutogenesis.'
(3) 'Application of a holistic and smooth therapeutic system with less side-effects, healing illness and imbalance through basic and repetitive improvements of self-regulating forces in the psychosomatic organism.'
(4) 'Criteria for the choice: (a) depends on pathology, (b) depends on patient choice, (c) less side-effects, (d) emergency (e.g. travelling tomorrow, antibiotics today).'
(5) 'Individual therapy – great respect for patient autonomy – "primum nil nocere" and to stimulate self-healing forces of the patient – synthesis of conventional primary care and complementary medicine – freedom of physician and patient.'

Wholeness: The Relational Dimension

The relational dimension of wholeness can be emphasized in a variety of ways, from a narrow focus on processes occurring during the consultation to a broader perspective of interconnectedness and 'togetherness' with others within the whole of nature and spiritual world [20].

Examples:

(1) 'First priority: listen, listen, listen. (2) Through specific questions complete details of case-taking. (3) Examine the patient, conventionally and with auricular diagnostics. (4) Share and discuss your impressions with the patient. (5) Discuss therapeutic options and propositions with the patient. (6) Begin the therapy. (7) Discuss further therapeutic options with the patient and understand her point of view. (8) Plan further steps. (9) Say good-bye to the patient.'
(2) 'The goal is to help the patient together with other stakeholders in the health care system, but the patient is the king!'
(3) 'From the human and relational point of view, the approach of complementary medicine is much more open, sincere and straight and therefore brings more satisfaction.'

Discussion

Dimensions of Holism: Relationship to Other Studies

Insights from qualitative and quantitative patient- and physician-related PEK data reveal the importance of holistic values and the multidimensionality of this concept. Accordingly, four interrelated dimensions of holism emerged: wholeness of patient, wholeness of physician, wholeness as integration and synthesis of conventional and complementary therapeutic approaches, the relational dimension (to the human, social, natural and spiritual environment). With respect to these dimensions, parallels to other studies exist.

Wholeness of patient: The importance and need to care and treat the 'whole person' is well documented in conventional primary care, is described and investigated from theoretical as well as empirical perspectives, and from the perspective of patients as well as physicians [3, 11, 12, 24, 31].

Relational dimension: Awareness of the relational aspect of holism in its broadest sense including religious and spiritual aspects characterizes both philosophical and CAM approaches to holism. This relational aspect encompasses 'interconnectedness between patient, practitioner and environment' [17], 'active participation in the whole, in the health and healing of the whole world' [4], the conviction that health of the parts and of the whole are interdependent [4], the 'togetherness' with the natural and social worlds [20]. Whereas philosophical and CAM approaches to holism rather emphasize the macrocosmic aspects of interconnectedness or the relationships between microcosm and macrocosm, the relational dimension of holism addressed in primary care seems to focus more on the patient-physician relationship and on communication including factors such as relational continuity and empathy [3, 12, 24].

Integration of therapeutic approaches: Integration of conventional and complementary medicine is a main characteristic of the CAM physicians that were assessed in PEK (and also of 15% of conventional physicians!) [2]. Confirming trends in the international literature [32–34], integration is a constant key feature in physicians' answers to all the questions (table 1) [2]. This increasing trend does not seem to be fully acknowledged by some authors writing on holism: 'While allopathic medicine recognises the complex interplay of these conditions, some alternative practitioners who claim to be holistic are in fact far more biologically reductionist' [11]. At the same time, holism and the hope for better health are associated with a combination of a variety of therapies, yet without mentioning complementary medicine [11]. Therefore, a holistic attitude that integrates different therapeutic approaches is not only a matter of medical practice, but also an attitude that acknowledges the reality of integrative medicine and the necessity to overcome the sometimes presumed incompatibility of conventional and complementary medicine as diametrically opposed practices and categories [4].

Wholeness of physician: In previous literature and as far as I am aware, physicians' satisfaction with their profession was either investigated in the context of complementary medicine or associated with holism. The broad and encompassing satisfaction with their profession documented by physicians who practise complementary medicine contrasts with the dissatisfaction of physicians as repeatedly demonstrated in public protests in the last years (e.g. in Germany, France and Switzerland). In the United States, physician health and wellness is addressed in the context of ethics policy and connected with the quality and safety of care. As the American Medical Association states, 'the medical profession has an obligation to ensure that its members are able to provide safe and effective care. This obligation is discharged by: promoting health and wellness among physicians' [35]. Such implications on quality of care should be taken into consideration and brought into balance when evaluating the benefits of complementary medicine.

Strengths and Weaknesses of this Study

This is one of only few studies on holism in the context of primary care integrating complementary medicine and including both patient and physician views.

Some weaknesses of this study are related to its methodology. The limitations of the PEK study on philosophy of care are described elsewhere [2]. These also apply to the present study. To explore holism, methods specifically used in qualitative research, e.g. interviews and focus groups, would have been more appropriate than questionnaires. Nevertheless, the broad spectrum of questions (table 1) has led to new insights and revealed possibilities how to interpret holism, e.g. by including the dimension of physician satisfaction, which adds a new aspect to current discussions. Physicians seem to experience satisfaction at different levels: with respect to philosophical and paradigmatic issues, medical practice, relationships and at a personal level. Nevertheless, the focus on the physician perspective in the 4-dimension model of holism could be completed and/or modified by including the perspective of patients.

Methodological Issues

Experiences and reflections linked to methodological issues arising in this article may contribute to the ongoing debate about appropriate research methodologies in CAM, particularly in the context of HTAs. Due to its political aims, the qualitative part of the PEK study (philosophy of care) was considered as less important with respect to the political decision than quantitative data which were expected to give rather definitive answers about perceived effectiveness and satisfaction of patients. Today, 2 years after the political decision about CAM, we may observe, first, that the huge amount of quantitative data collected was ignored by the responsible authorities as soon as these data revealed results in favour of complementary medicine. Second, after the political decision of 2005, scientific work on PEK data was further associated with power games, arbitrariness and a lack of fairness given the concentration of power related to the ownership, administration and management of PEK data. Third, quantitative data have to be reflected, interpreted and understood. In particular, an interpretation and understanding of the EUROPEP results (European Task Force on Patient Evaluation of Practice [36, 37]) to my knowledge has not yet been convincingly addressed. These results suggest better satisfaction of patients with physicians who integrate complementary and conventional medicine. Forth, investigating philosophical issues (empirically or conceptually) may be as important and relevant for health policy as quantitative assessments. Thus, such observations confirm previous research [21] on the importance to integrate philosophical issues into HTAs and to acknowledge their actuality and potential. Furthermore, combining quantitative and qualitative approaches, such as in PEK, and completing them by further theoretical and conceptual work is a 'holistic' way appropriate to the complexity of complementary medicine.

Linking Holism and Patient Satisfaction

Further, I would like to make a link between a holistic approach on the one side and the PEK results concerning better satisfaction with complementary than conventional care on the other side [1].

Holism is increasingly been recognised as a core element of general practice. The PEK studies show that holism is an essential part of physicians' philosophy of care in complementary medicine. Furthermore, the PEK studies also suggest that holism is one of the most important reasons for choosing a physician of complementary medicine [1, 2].
Recent developments and discussions in primary care suggest an increasing importance of holism as well as the importance of changes. Reflecting on the PEK results we may ask if some of these changes and developments are anticipated or partly realised by complementary medicine and if this contributes to the high satisfaction of patients with a model of care that integrates conventional and complementary approaches. Olesen et al. [38], for example, suggest that it is time for general practice to revise the academic agenda and to incorporate more insights from behavioural sciences into the undergraduate curriculum and specialist trainings. According to a current definition of general practice the 'general practitioner engages with autonomous individuals across the fields of prevention, diagnosis, cure, and palliation, using and integrating the sciences of biomedicine, medical psychology and medical sociology' [38]. Even though medical sociology and psychology are not explicitly cited in the philosophy of care of CAM physicians, the philosophical background of CAM disciplines (e.g. anthroposophic medicine, homeopathy, traditional Chinese medicine) may lead to a particular awareness of psychological and social problems. Homeopathic treatment, for example, is based on a detailed case-taking including all reported or observed symptoms of the patient's body and personality as well as physical, emotional, social and spiritual aspects [13, 39, 40]. In further research, it would also be interesting to consider patient satisfaction with complementary medicine on the background of the virtue approach to medical ethics [31]. Possibly, the philosophical frameworks of some complementary disciplines may also contribute to developing moral virtues associated with the practice of medicine. These have been neglected in medical education which is still focusing too much on the natural sciences [3, 31].
The reason for higher satisfaction with care, especially regarding communication, as reflected by the results of the satisfaction survey EUROPEP [1], may be seen in this context, too. It is noticeable that in the discussion on holism in primary care, the aspects mentioned are related to communication in the broadest sense and that in the PEK studies, these were rated significantly better in complementary medicine than in conventional primary care [1]. Therefore, the relationship between the holistic approach of physicians and patient satisfaction needs further research. If holism is increasingly recognised as core dimension in primary care and seems to be realised in an integrative approach such as that assessed in PEK, why should it not be worthy of reimbursement in basic insurance, as it was decided by the Swiss Minister of Health in 2005?

Further Sub-Themes, Implications and Research Questions
Further sub-themes that emerge from the data and are of importance for society as a whole are gender and environmental issues. There is increasing evidence for gender-related differences and bias in academic and clinical medicine [41, 42]. Against this background, the fact that complementary medicine is practised and used more often by women, as suggested by quantitative and qualitative data of PEK as well as CAM research in general, could also be further discussed in the context of holism.
A therapeutic attitude that is respectful of the environment is a further theme emerging from philosophy of care of physicians practising complementary medicine and is related to current challenges concerning society and humankind as a whole. Like the gender issues, this awareness of ecological issues found among CAM physicians could also be further investigated in the context of holism.

Conclusion

Insights won from qualitative and quantitative, patient and physician PEK data reveal the importance of holistic values and the multidimensionality of the concept. If understood this way, a holistic approach to health and medicine is in accordance with current developments and discussions about core values and aims of primary care. Therefore, such an integrative approach should be acknowledged with respect to consequences for quality of care, policy and educational issues.

Acknowledgements

I thank Hans-Ueli Albonico, André Thurneysen, Klaus von Ammon and Peter Heusser for their support and helpful discussions. This study was supported by the Merkur-Rafael Foundation, by the Fondation Homéopathique Pierre Schmidt and the University of Bern. I thank Harald Walach for his review of the manuscript.

References

1 Melchart D, Mitscherlich F, Amiet M, Eichenberger R, Koch P: Programm Evaluation Komplementärmedizin (PEK), Schlussbericht. Bern, Bundesamt für Gesundheit, 2005.
2 Marian F, Widmer M, Herren S, Donges A, Busato A: Physicians' philosophy of care: a comparison of complementary and conventional medicine. Forsch Komplementärmed 2006;13:70–77.
3 Strandberg EL, Ovhed I, Borgquist L, Wilhelmsson S: The perceived meaning of a (w)holistic view among general practitioners and district nurses in Swedish primary care: a qualitative study. BMC Fam Pract 2007;8:8.
4 Walach H: [On the path to complete health]. Forsch Komplementärmed Klass Naturheilkd 2003; 10:5–6.
5 Boyd KM: Disease, illness, sickness, health, healing and wholeness: exploring some elusive concepts. Med Humanities 2000;26:9–17.
6 Bensing J: Bridging the gap. The separate worlds of evidence-based medicine and patient-centred medicine. Patient Educ Couns 2000;39:17–25.

7 Stempsey W: Plato and holistic medicine. Med Health Care Philosophy 2001;4:201.
8 Moravcsik J: Health, healing, and Plato's ethics. J Value Inquiry 2000;34:7–26.
9 Plato: The Collected Dialogues of Plato. New Jersey, Princeton University Press, 1989.
10 Benaroyo L: Ethique et responsabilité en médecine. Genève, Médecine et hygiène, 2006.
11 Freeman J: Towards a definition of holism. Br J Gen Pract 2005;55:154–155.
12 Tarrant C, Windridge K, Boulton M, Baker R, Freeman G: How important is personal care in general practice? BMJ 2003;326:1310.
13 Kaptchuk TJ, Eisenberg DM: The persuasive appeal of alternative medicine. Ann Intern Med 1998; 129:1061–1065.
14 Barrett B, Marchand L, Scheder J, Plane MB, Maberry R, Appelbaum D, Rakel D, Rabago D: Themes of holism, empowerment, access, and legitimacy define complementary, alternative, and integrative medicine in relation to conventional biomedicine. J Altern Complement Med 2003;9:937–947.
15 Saks M: Alternative therapies: are they holistic? Complement Ther Nurs Midwifery 1997;3:4–8.
16 Meyer-Abich KM: [How holistic is health? – from Hippocrates and Plato to a future sociopsychosomatic situational therapy]. Forsch Komplementärmed Klass Naturheilkd 2003;10:35–39.
17 Long AF: Outcome measurement in complementary and alternative medicine: unpicking the effects. J Altern Complement Med 2002;8:777–786.
18 Astin JA: Why patients use alternative medicine: results of a national study. JAMA 1998;279: 1548–1553.
19 Bishop FL, Yardley L, Lewith G: Developing a measure of treatment beliefs: the complementary and alternative medicine beliefs inventory. Complement Ther Med 2005;13:144–149.
20 Meyer-Abich KM: [The meaning of wholeness in medical philosophy.]. Forsch Komplementärmed 2007;14:240–246.
21 Verhoef MJ, Vanderheyden LC, Dryden T, Mallory D, Ware MA: Evaluating complementary and alternative medicine interventions: in search of appropriate patient-centered outcome measures. BMC Complement Altern Med 2006;6:6–38.
22 Lawrence C, Weisz G: Greater than the parts: holism in biomedicine 1920–1950. New York, Oxford University Press, 1998.
23 Goldstein MS, Sutherland CE, Jaffe DT, Wilson J: Holistic physicians and family practitioners: an empirical comparison. Fam Med 1987;19:281–286.
24 Mercer S, Cawston P, Bikker A: Quality in general practice consultations; a qualitative study of the views of patients living in an area of high socio-economic deprivation in Scotland. BMC Family Pract 2007;8:22.
25 Marian F, Albonico H-U, Heusser P, Busato A: Evaluation of anthroposophic medicine in Switzerland: structures, procedures and outcomes of care. Bern, Bundesamt für Gesundheit, 2005.
26 Heusser P: PEK und BAG: Probleme beim Programm Evaluation Komplementärmedizin. Schweiz Ärzteztg 2006;87:899–903.
27 Heusser P: Medizin und Macht am Beispiel des Programms Evaluation Komplementärmedizin PEK; in Ausfeld-Hafter B (Hrsg): Medizin und Macht. Die Arzt-Patienten-Beziehung im Wandel: mehr Entscheidungsfreiheit? Bern, Peter Lang, 2007.
28 Walach H, Linde K, Eichenberger R, Stalder H, Borlum Kristensen F, Kleijnen J: Summary consensus statement of the Review Board of the Swiss Complementary Medicine Evaluation Programme, (Programme Evaluation Komplementarmedizin, PEK) regarding the PEK process and products. Homeopathy 2006;95:28–30.
29 Walach H: The Swiss program for the evaluation of complementary medicine (PEK). J Altern Complement Med 2006;12:231–232.
30 Moustakas C: Phenomenological research methods. Thousand Oaks, Sage, 1994.
31 Braunack-Mayer A: What makes a good GP? An empirical perspective on virtue in general practice. J Med Ethics 2005;31:82–87.
32 Berman BM: Integrative approaches to pain management: how to get the best of both worlds. BMJ 2003;326:1320-a-1321.
33 Bodeker G: Lessons on integration from the developing world's experience. BMJ 2001;322:164–167.
34 Kaptchuk TJ, Miller FG: Viewpoint: what is the best and most ethical model for the relationship between mainstream and alternative medicine: opposition, integration, or pluralism? Acad Med 2005; 80:286–290.
35 American Medical Association (ed): AMA Ethics Policy. E-90305 Physician Health and Wellness. American Medical Association, 2007.
36 Grol R, Wensing M, Mainz J, Ferreira P, Hearnshaw H, Hjortdahl P, Olesen F, Ribacke M, Spenser T, Szecsenyi J: Patients' priorities with respect to general practice care: an international comparison. European Task Force on Patient Evaluations of General Practice (EUROPEP). Fam Pract 1999;16: 4–11.
37 Grol R, Wensing M, Mainz J, Jung HP, Ferreira P, Hearnshaw H, Hjortdahl P, Olesen F, Reis S, Ribacke M, Szecsenyi J: Patients in Europe evaluate general practice care: an international comparison. Br J Gen Pract 2000;50:882–887.
38 Olesen F, Dickinson J, Hjortdahl P: General practice – time for a new definition. BMJ 2000;320: 354–357.
39 Rabovsky K: Homöopathie und ärztliche Ethik – Begriffe und handlungsorientierende Werte homöopathischer Ärzte heute. Institut für Geschichte der Medizin, Medizinische Fakultät. Freiburg i.Br., Albert-Ludwigs-Universität, 1993.
40 Thompson TD, Weiss M: Homeopathy – what are the active ingredients? An exploratory study using the UK Medical Research Council's framework for the evaluation of complex interventions. BMC Complement Altern Med 2006;6:37.
41 Doyal L: Gender equity in health: debates and dilemmas. Soc Sci Med 2000;51:931.
42 Risberg G, Johansson E, Westman G, Hamberg K: Gender in medicine – an issue for women only? A survey of physician teachers' gender attitudes. Int J Equity Health 2003;2:10.

Forschende Komplementärmedizin
Wissenschaft • Praxis • Perspektiven

Guidelines for Authors

Forsch Komplementärmed 2007;14

Submission

'Research in Complementary Medicine' is a peer-reviewed journal that publishes articles written in German or English on basic research, clinical studies, methodology or scientific theory in complementary medicine.
Manuscripts can be submitted online at *www.karger.com/fok.*
Should you have any problems with electronic submission, please contact the Editorial Office:

S. Karger Verlag für Medizin und Naturwissenschaften GmbH
Attn.: Dipl.-Psych. Franziska Lang
P.O. Box
79095 Freiburg (Germany)
Tel. +49 761 45 20 726
Fax +49 761 45 20 714
E-mail f.lang@karger.de

Types of Papers and Allotted Number of Pages

Manuscripts should be written double-spaced, 12-point size, with 3-cm margins. Please use only one format (normal) for the document.
Contributions are classified as: Original Article, Review Article, Case Report, Essay, Methodology, Documentation, Editorial, Journal Club, Congress Report, Book Review, Letter to the Editors. Articles should not exceed 8 printed pages (case reports: 4). Short communications of scientific results should not exceed 3 printed pages. (As a rule of thumb, 3 manuscript pages, including cover sheet, tables, figures are equal to 1 printed page.) Each additional complete or partial page to print will be charged to the author.

Reports on Randomized Controlled Trials (RCTs) should be prepared according to the CONSORT statement [Begg C, Cho M, Eastwood S, Horton S, Moher D, Olki I, Pitkin R, Rennie D, Schulz F, Simel D, Stroup D: Improving the quality of reporting of randomized trials: The CONSORT statement. JAMA 1996;276:637–639]. The report must state explicitly how the comparison groups were assembled, allowing the reader to access the method of randomization. Please specify in the title and summary that the manuscript is a report on an RCT. When an RCT is submitted, the authors should refer to the 'Checklist for Authors Submitting Randomized Controlled Trials' available at *http://www.consort-statement.org*. Both should be submitted with the manuscript, as they will be included in the review process.
Reports on homeopathic treatments should be prepared according to the RedHot-Supplement to CONSORT [Dean ME, Coulter MK, Fisher P, Jobst K, Walach H: Reporting data on homeopathic treatments (RedHot): A supplement to CONSORT. Forsch Komplementärmed 2006;13:368–371].

Conditions

Acceptance of a manuscript is based on the evaluation by several reviewers (peer review).
Manuscripts are received with the explicit understanding that they are not under simultaneous consideration by any other publication. Submission of an article for publication implies the transfer of the copyright from the author to the publisher upon acceptance.
Once the manuscript is accepted for publication, all usage rights will be retained by the publisher. The assignment of usage rights applies to all print media as well as electronic offline and online media, including the Internet and data bases/data carriers of any kind. Accepted papers, in whole or in part, may not be translated into other languages, or reproduced by any mechanical or electronic means (including photocopying, recording and microcopying), or stored in a retrieval system without the written consent of the publisher.
It is the authors' responsibility to obtain permission to produce illustrations, tables, etc. from other publications.
All forms of support, including that from drug companies, and any potential source of conflict of interest should be acknowledged in the cover letter to the editor. Should the manuscript be accepted, the editor will discuss the extent of disclosure appropriate for publication with the authors. The publisher reserves the right to edit the manuscript and decide on the layout.

Ethical and Legal Prerequisites

Manuscripts involving examinations of probands and patents must include a statement that the trial protocol has been approved by an ethical committee and thus meets the standards of the Declaration of Helsinki in its revised version of 1975 and its amendments of 1983, 1989, and 1996 [JAMA 1997;277:925–926]. Accordingly, the proband's informed consent has to be mentioned in the manuscript. Information suitable to reveal the proband's identity is to be avoided.
Experiments involving animals demand consent as well and must meet the requirements of German laws for the protection of animals in their current version. A reference to this approval must be included in the manuscript. Articles from countries other than Germany must include a comparable note.

Arrangement

Authors' affiliations and address of correspondence: Each author's full name, followed by their affiliation (hospital, institute etc. where the work was conducted) and the exact postal address of the corresponding author must be given in a separate document to allow a blind review process. Please also supply phone and fax numbers, as well as e-mail address.

Title page: The first page of each paper should indicate the title (in German **and** English) and a short title for use as running head.

Key Words: For indexing purposes, a list of 3–5 key words in English and German is essential. Whenever possible, use key words such as found in the Medical Subject Headings List (MeSH) of Index Medicus.

Summary: Summaries must be submitted in German and English. They must not exceed 250 words each. Summaries of Original Articles should be structured as follows: Background (or Introduction), Patients and Methods (or Material and Methods), Results, Conclusion.

Footnotes: Footnotes should be used only for tables.

Registered Trade Names: When first mentioned, registered trade names must be marked with the superscript registration symbol ® or TM. It is the sole responsibility of the author to ensure that this rule is followed properly.

Tables and Illustrations: Tables and illustrations should be prepared on separate sheets. *Tables* require a heading and figures a legend, also prepared on a separate sheet. The number of figures and tables should be limited and aim to illustrate the text. Figures are listed in the text as (fig. 1), tables as (table 1). Data already mentioned in the text need not be repeated in a table. Accordingly, numbers used in tables need not be repeated in the text.
For the reproduction of *illustrations*, only good drawings and original photographs can be accepted. On the back of each illustration, indicate its number, the author's name, and 'top' with a soft pencil. Electronically submitted b/w half-tone and color illustrations must have a final resolution of 300 dpi after scaling, line drawings one of 800–1200 dpi.
Color illustrations are reproduced at the author's expense. Each one is charged to the author at EUR 270.– + VAT as contribution to the additional reproduction and color printing costs.

References

The list of **references** should include only the publications cited in the text. References must be numbered sequentially in the order cited in the text. In the text identify references by Arabic numerals [in square brackets]. In each reference at least the first 3 authors should be named. It is recommended to quote only articles already published or accepted for publication. Please avoid 'in preparation' or 'personal communication'. Authors are responsible for the accuracy and completeness of their references and for correct citation. Journal titles should be abbreviated according to the Index Medicus system (www.nlm.nih.gov). If a reference manager is used, the style «Pharmacology» or «Nephron» should be chosen.
Examples for references:

Papers published in periodicals:
1 Lelie PN, Cuypers HTM, van Drimmelen AAJ, Quint WGV: Quality assessment of hepatitis C virus nucleic acid amplification methods. An international proficiency study. Infusionsther Transfusionsmed 1998;25:102–110.

Papers published only with DOI numbers:
2 Theoharides TC, Boucher W, Spear K: Serum interleukin-6 reflects disease severity and osteoporosis in mastocytosis patients. Int Arch Allergy Immunol DOI: 10.1159/000063858.

Papers published in electronic format:
3 Black CA: Delayed type hypersensitivity: Current theories with a historic perspective. Dermatol Online J 1999;5:7. http://dermatology.dclib.org/DOJvol5num1.

Edited books:
4 Hardy WD Jr, Essex M: FeLV-induced feline acquired immune deficiency syndrome: A model for human AIDS; in Klein E (ed): Acquired Immunodeficiency Syndrome. Prog Allergy. Basel, Karger, 1986, vol 37, pp 353–376.

Monographs:
5 Schaefer UW, Beelen DW: Bone Marrow Transplantation, ed 2, revised. Basel, Karger, 1996.

Page Charges

There are no page charges for papers that do not exceed the allotted size (cf. types of papers). Each additional complete or partial page is charged to the author at 380.– EUR + VAT.

Galley Proofs

Unless indicated otherwise, galley proofs are sent to the corresponding author and should be returned with the least possible delay. Alterations made in galley proofs, other than the correction of printer's errors, are charged to the author. No page proofs are supplied.

Reprints

Order forms and a price list are sent with the galley proofs. Orders submitted after the issue is printed are subject to considerably higher prices.

KARGER
Fax +49 761 4 52 07 14
E-mail Information@Karger.de
www.karger.com

Guidelines for Authors available at:
www.karger.com/fok_gl.htm